STOP THE ROLLERCOASTER

HOW TO TAKE CHARGE OF YOUR BLOOD SUGARS IN DIABETES

By

John Walsh, P.A., C.D.E.

Ruth Roberts, M.A.

Lois Jovanovic-Peterson, M.D.

Plus "Charting With Computers" by Timothy S. Bailey, M.D., F.A.C.P., F.A.C.E.

Torrey Pines Press
1030 West Upas Street
San Diego, California 92103-3821
1-800-988-4772
1-619-497-0900

Library of Congress Cataloging in Publication Data

STOP The Rollercoaster
    How To Take Charge Of Your Blood Sugars In Diabetes
    John Walsh, P.A., C.D.E., Ruth Roberts, M.A., and Lois Jovanovic-Peterson, M.D.

1996
230 pages
166 bibliographical references.
Index.
1. Diabetes-Popular Works
      i. Walsh, John
      ii. Roberts, Ruth
      iii. Jovanovic-Peterson, Lois
2. Diabetes--Insulin
3. Diabetes--Insulin-dependent diabetes
4. Diabetes--Research
5. Insulin--Therapeutic use
I. Title

ISBN 1-884804-82-9 $21.95   Paperback

Printed in the United States of America 2 3 4 5 6 7 8 9 0

WHAT PEOPLE ARE SAYING

"If Forrest Gump were diabetic, his mamma might have said, 'Blood sugars are like a box of chocolate. You never know what you're going to get.' For you riders of inexplicable blood sugar climbs and plunges, help is here.

Nothing hit or miss about this book. Detailed training in matching doses to food and exercise; adjusting for highs, lows and emergencies; charting blood sugars; and even in handling costs. If you've been flying your blood sugars by the seat of your pants, this book is like getting an advanced instrument system and radar to guide you."

June Biermann and Barbara Toobey
Prolific authors of books and newsletters for people with diabetes.

"Did you ever wish your diabetes came with an owner's manual? Now you can have one, if you are on a multiple injection regimen or thinking about it. After years of recommending *Pumping Insulin* to pumpers and people interested in pumping, I can now recommend *Stop the Rollercoaster* with as much confidence and enthusiasm to everyone with diabetes. This book fills a long-standing empty space on the diabetes bookshelf."

Joan Stout
Durham, North Carolina

"This book is packed full of information—sort of like a 'nutrient-rich' compendium for people using insulin. For practical management of insulin, if you can't find your answer here, you probably won't find it anywhere."

Claudia Graham, C.D.E., Ph.D., M.P.H.
Consultive Physiologist and Director of Managed Care for VIVRA Health Advantage,
Los Angeles, California

"*Stop the Rollercoaster* is a practical tool for motivated insulin users, which will enhance the participation in their own diabetes management. As a diabetes health care provider, I will certainly help my patients individualize the suggestions presented to improve their blood glucose control."

Evelyne Fleury-Milfort, M.S.N., C-R.N.P., C.D.E.
Program Coordinator, USC Center for Diabetes, Los Angeles, California

"Personally, the techniques taught in this book have helped me to achieve eight years of excellent diabetes control while living a flexible, vaired and active lifestyle. Professionally, the excellent charts, graphs, and step by step instructions have enabled me to teach others to achieve the same goals. If these are *your* goals, then this is the book for you."

JoAnne Scott, R.N., B.S.N., C.D.E.
Spokane, Washington

"Insulin was discovered 70 years ago. *Finally*, this book gives the directions to use it to achieve good control and health."

Alan O. Marcus, M.D., F.A.C.P.
Associate Clinical Professor, U.S.C. School of Medicine

An Important Note

    Stop the Rollercoaster has been developed as a guide. Guidelines, examples, situations and sample charts are included to provide basic and advanced information related to the use of flexible insulin therapy. *Insulin requirements and treatment protocols differ significantly from one person to the next.* The information included in this book should be used only as a guide. It is not a substitute for the sound medical advice of your personal physician/health care team. Treatment plans, insulin dosages and other aspects of health care for a person with diabetes must be individualized under the guidance of your physician/health care team. The information in this book is provided to enhance your understanding of diabetes so that you can manage the daily lifestyle challenges you face. It can never be relied upon as a sole source for your personal diabetes regimen.

    While every reasonable precaution has been taken in the preparation of this information, the authors and publishers assume no responsibility for errors or omissions, nor for the uses made of the materials contained herein and the decisions based on such use. No warranties are made, expressed or implied, with regard to the contents of this work or to its applicability to specific individuals. The authors and publishers shall not be liable for direct, indirect, special, incidental, or consequential damages arising out of the use of or inability to use the contents of this book.

ABOUT THE AUTHORS

John Walsh has worked as a Physician Assistant and provided comprehensive patient care as a diabetes clinical specialist for 15 years. Drawing from his personal and professional experience with diabetes, he has given numerous presentations to physicians, health professionals and private groups, including the American Diabetes Association, Juvenile Diabetes Foundation, International Diabetic Athletes Association, and a variety of hospital and support groups.

He received the 1993 O. Charles Olson Lectureship Award and is a member of the board of directors of the International Diabetic Athletes Association. He has authored or co-authored several dozen articles and research papers and three books on insulin pump therapy. He is a columnist for *Diabetes Interview* and has been a repeat guest on the national radio and TV programs "Living With Diabetes." He is recognized as an innovator in diabetes control and the prevention of complications. He lives in San Diego.

Ruth Roberts is a corporate training administrator, technical/medical writer, and instructional designer in San Diego. She has been involved in diabetes support groups for over ten years and co-authored, *Pumping Insulin*, the *Diabetes Advanced Workbook* and the *Insulin Pump Therapy Handbook*. Ruth has written the "PumpFormance" column in *Diabetes Interview* and has been a guest on "Living With Diabetes" as an educational expert on intensive self-management. She is a professional member of the American Diabetes Association, the American Association of Diabetes Educators and past Program Director of the San Diego Chapter of the American Society for Training and Development.

Lois Jovanovic-Peterson, M.D. is a senior scientist at the Sansum Medical Research Foundation in Santa Barbara. She is a board certified internist and endocrinologist and is the current president of the California Affiliate of the American Diabetes Association. She has served as the chair of the Pregnancy Council of the American Diabetes Association. She has received the Clintec Award for Excellence in the field of nutrition from the American College of Nutrition, and the Soroptomist International Award for Excellence in the field of medicine.

Her research interests have been in the fields of diabetes and pregnancy and islet cell transplantation. Because of her international acclaim in the field of diabetes and pregnancy, she was elected an Honorary Member by the European Association for the Study of Diabetes, the only member from the United States and only the 12th in the world with this honor! She was named the American Diabetes Association's Outstanding Physician Clinician for 1995 in tribute to her many contributions in diabetes.

Lois is one of the earliest advocates for direct involvement of the individual who has diabetes with his or her own blood sugar management. She and her husband, Dr. Charles M. Peterson, have been pioneers in the use of intensified insulin delivery systems for pregnant women with diabetes. She has authored hundreds of articles on the topic of diabetes, and authored or co-authored 24 books on diabetes, including many on the management of the pregnant and non-pregnant diabetic woman. The challenge and struggle with her own diabetes also has prepared her to present the materials in this book.

Timothy Bailey, M.D., F.A.C.P., F.A.C.E., is an assistant clincial professor of medicine at the University of California, San Diego, School of Medicine. He is a clinical endrocrinologist in private practice in San Diego and head of MetaMedix™, a company that produces diabetes management aids and computer software.

DEDICATION

This book is for John and Ruth's parents:
    Jack and Katie Walsh, and
    Bessie and P.C. Roberts.

Lois Jovanovic-Peterson, M.D. wishes to thank
    her soul mate, best friend and husband, Charles M. Peterson, M.D.,
    and her loving children, Kevin, Larisa and Boyce.

ACKNOWLEDGMENTS

Stop the Rollercoaster is the product of many years of personal and professional experience with diabetes. The authors have a total of 85 years of personal experience with diabetes and 40 years of clinical and research experience. During this time, major contributions have been made by our patients, friends, family members, colleagues, and fellow travelers in meeting the challenges of diabetes.

Our heartfelt thanks goes to the following people:

Bessie Roberts of La Grange, Kentucky; Patricia and Kathryn Greten of San Diego; JoAnne Scott, R.N., C.D.E., and Jeffrey Hartman, M.D., in private practice in Spokane, Washington; June Biermann and Barbara Toohey, authors of books and newsletters for people with diabetes, of Van Nuys, California; Evelyne Fleury-Milfort, R.N.P., C.D.E.,of the USC Center for Diabetes, Los Angeles; Claudia Graham, C.D.E., M.P.H., Ph.D., of VIVRA Health Advantage, Los Angeles; Scott King of *Diabetes Interview*, San Francisco; Carol Wysham, M.D., of the Rockwood Clinic, Spokane, Washington; Marilyn James, management systems consultant of Del Mar, Calif.; Timothy Bailey, M.D., F.A.C.P., of North County Endocrinology, Escondido, California; and Alan Marcus, M.D., F.A.C.P., of South Orange County Endocrinology, Laguna Hills, California, who graciously and critically reviewed and improved upon this book.

The American Diabetes Association; the Juvenile Diabetes Foundation; the National Institute of Health; and other national agencies that have generously supported diabetes education and research.

All the health practitioners and the 1,441 volunteers with diabetes who participated in the Diabetes Control and Complications Trial. This historic study (which confirmed what many already assumed--that controlling blood sugars reduces the complications of diabetes) laid the groundwork for this book on taking control of your blood sugars.

Paula Harper and the International Diabetic Athletes Association for providing international conferences and a newsletter where we presented ideas and received feedback from people with diabetes who exercise. In this highly interactive and enjoyable forum, we developed the information on exercise over the past few years.

Michelle R. Hays of Visual Designs, San Diego, who created the marvelous cover and chapter headings;

Joan Stout of Durham, North Carolina, who enthusiastically and laboriously generated the index;

Kevin Ansberry of Dublin, California, for his delightful cartoons and illustrations which lightened the intensity of this information and often communicated the message in a way that facts and words on their own can't; and

Karen Boyd of San Diego for excellence in editing, organizing and clarifying during these last few weeks just when we thought we would go crazy on our own.

Other books by John Walsh, P.A., C.D.E. and Ruth Roberts, M.A.:

Pocket Pancreas, *Torrey Pines Press, 1995*
Pumping Insulin, *second edition, Torrey Pines Press, 1994*
Insulin Pump Therapy Handbook, *MiniMed Technologies, 1990*
Pumping Insulin, *first editon, MiniMed Technologies, 1989*
Diabetes Advanced Workbook, *1988*

Other books by Lois Jovanovic-Peterson, M.D.:

Endocrine Disorders of Pregnancy, Endocrine Clinics of North America, *W.B. Saunders, 1995,*
    edited with Charles M. Peterson, M.D.
Gestational Diabetes, *DCI Publishing, 1994, with M. B. Stone*
Medical Management of Pregnancy Complicated by Diabetes, *American Diabetes Association,*
    1993, Editor-In-Chief
A Woman's Guide to Menopause, *Hyperion, 1993, with S. Levert*
A Touch of Diabetes, *DCI Publishing, 1991, with Charles M. Peterson, M.D.*
The Diabetes Self-Care Method, *Lowell House, 1990, edited with Charles M. Peterson, M.D.*
Controversies in the Field of Pregnancy and Diabetes, *Springer-Verlag, 1988, editor*
Hormones: The Woman's Answer Book, *Atheneum Publishers, 1987, with G. J. Subak-Sharpe*
    (French and German translations)
The Diabetic Woman, *Jeremy Tarcher Publishers, 1987, with June Bierman and Barbara*
    Toohey
Diabetes in Pregnancy: Teratology, Toxicology, and Treatment, *Praeger, 1986, edited with*
    Charles M. Peterson, M.D.
Contemporary Issues in Nutrition: Diabetes Mellitus, *Alan Liss, 1985, edited with Charles M.*
    Peterson, M.D.

TABLE OF CONTENTS

A Special Note to Readers

In addition to publishing books on diabetes care, Torrey Pines Press also offers products to help people better manage their diabetes. Three new products that may be of interest to our readers are introduced in *Stop the Rollercoaster.*

One is "The Blood Sugar Inventory and Action Guides" described in Chapter 5. The Inventory enables the person with diabetes to recognize areas where blood sugar control could be improved. Then the Action Guides provide suggestions for improving these trouble spots.

The second new item is the "Smart Charts," described in Chapter 6. These pocket-sized graphic charts offer an easy way to see at a glance a total daily record of carbs eaten, insulin taken, blood sugar readings and events that affect the blood sugar.

The third is Mellitus Manager®, a software program that can be used with meters to download the data gathered into a computer, and analyze it through charts and graphs. This allows the data to be used to improve blood sugar control.

If, after reading these chapters, you decide you would like the Blood Sugar Inventory and Action Guides (sold as one), a supply of Smart Charts, or the Mellitus Manager software, information for ordering each can be found at the back of this book.

Read This!

Never use this book on your own! Any suggestion made in this book for improving blood sugar control with flexible insulin therapy should be followed only with the approval and guidance of your personal physician.

We have provided the best information and tools available so that flexible insulin therapy can do its job of normalizing your blood sugars. The tools in this book have been developed and refined over almost two decades of clinical care, research and study in the diabetes health care field. They also draw on more than four decades of two of the authors' personal experience with their own diabetes. Several thousand people have improved their blood sugars and HbA_{1c} results by applying these tools.

But this book is not enough. We have worked with people who have used this information under the guidance of their physician and they have excelled. We have also seen people harm themselves by a selective use of this and other material, or by ignoring or not seeking excellent medical advice.

Always seek the advice and guidance of your physician and health care team. No book can ever help you as much as they will. They have experience gained from working with many individuals. Keep in mind the importance of good professional advice and support. Teams win where individuals fail, and teamwork takes trust and communication from everyone.

**We wish all of our readers the best in health
and control with their diabetes!**

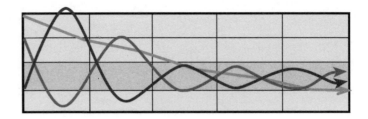

Do You Need This Book?

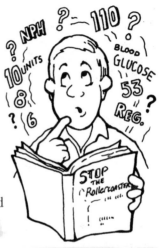

You may be wondering if this book can help you. You may have questions like: "Why are my blood sugars going up and down?" or "How do I know when my insulin doses need changing?" If blood sugar control and the use of insulin are some of your concerns about your diabetes, this book will provide you an in-depth outline for success. It can help anyone who wants to participate in taking charge of their own blood sugars.

Stop the Rollercoaster is for:

- Everyone who wants an end to highs and lows
- Anyone considering or beginning a program of improved blood sugar management as recommended by the Diabetes Control and Complications Trial (DCCT)
- Anyone now using flexible management who wants to improve their control
- The physicians, nurses, dieticians, physician assistants, nurse practitioners, and others who help improve their clients' health with diabetes

It can help you:

- Regulate your insulin doses through flexible insulin therapy
- Live a more varied life with better control
- Chart and analyze blood sugar tests
- Manage low blood sugars
- Manage high blood sugars
- Know when to get help
- Feel better and live a longer, healthier life.

Stop the Rollercoaster is organized into seven sections with related chapters. The book also has a glossary, an index, checklists for improving control, many step-by-step directions, and specific examples of management strategies. Included are three of the newest and most advanced blood sugar charting methods, comprehensive approaches to exercise and pregnancy, and information on the latest research and therapies for complications. If all of this sounds like information you can use, then read on.

LEARNING ABOUT DIABETES

CHAPTER 1.   WHY KEEP BLOOD SUGARS NORMAL?

CHAPTER 2.   TYPES OF DIABETES AND HOW TREATMENT
DIFFERS

CHAPTER 3.   CAN FLEXIBLE INSULIN THERAPY HELP YOU?

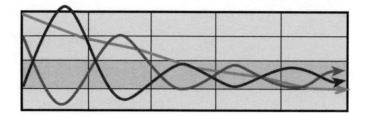

WHY KEEP BLOOD SUGARS NORMAL?

1

When you have diabetes you may sometimes wonder, "Will I ever be able to live a normal life?" We are happy to report that tens of thousands of people with diabetes have had enough information and determination to come darn close.

Learning to control blood sugars and faithfully carrying out the appropriate actions for your health is often a real challenge! In fact, keeping blood sugars near normal is the greatest challenge you face with diabetes.

The whole purpose of this book is to provide you with the information, tools and motivation needed to take on this challenge and succeed. In this chapter, we will look at some of the reasons you will want to accept this challenge. In future chapters, we provide practical ways to successfully meet the challenge.

In this chapter, we'll discuss:

- Benefits of controlling the blood sugar
- How high blood sugars can cause complications
- Ways to prevent these complications

BENEFITS OF A NORMAL BLOOD SUGAR

Blood sugars that are too high can lead to damage in important cells and organs in the body. Nerve, eye and kidney cells are especially prone to the negative effect of high blood sugars. One clear benefit of keeping sugars normal is a lower risk for developing the serious complications of diabetes, such as kidney failure or blindness.

Research also suggests that normal blood sugars may protect against cardiovascular problems, such as heart attacks and strokes. People with diabetes are normally at higher risk for heart disease, in large part because of too many high sugars. Other risk factors for cardiovascular disease, like obesity and high blood pressure, are often associated with diabetes. Current research studies overwhelmingly show that *all the complications of diabetes can be prevented or lessened* if blood sugars are kept normal.

We will look at these conditions more closely in future chapters of this book. Our purpose here is to give you a simple, overall view of the importance of near-normal, stable blood sugars. How to achieve this with a flexible lifestyle is the theme of *Stop the Rollercoaster*.

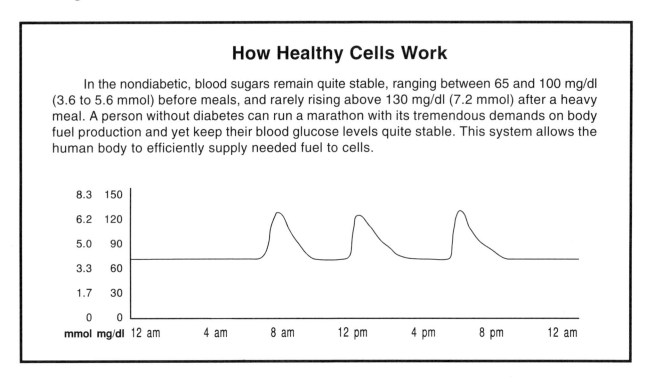

Figure 1.1 Normal blood sugar pattern in a person who eats three meals a day

DCCT: Normal Blood Sugars Lower the Risk of Complications

One of those most important studies of diabetes in recent years has provided invaluable information on the benefits of normal blood sugars. The Diabetes Control and Complications Trial (DCCT) is an exciting nine-year study that cost $167 million.

In the study, a group of 1,441 people with Type I diabetes were followed for three to nine years. Half were randomly assigned to a "control" group in which blood sugars were *conventionally controlled* on one or two injections a day. The other half were assigned to an *intensive control* group with the task of keeping their blood sugars as normal as possible using three or more injections a day (or insulin pumps).

Compared to the conventional control group, the intensive control group experienced *up to 76 percent less eye damage, 54 percent less kidney disease and 60 percent less neuropathy.*[1]

As you can see by these findings, the study proved beyond a doubt that people who intensively control their blood sugars have less risk of complications. Many researchers had long suspected this was true. But the exciting finding of the DCCT was how much these complications were eliminated.[1]

Although this study was carried out with subjects having Type I diabetes, most diabetes specialists feel the same conclusions about control can be drawn for people with Type II diabetes. *High blood sugars create damage no matter what type of diabetes is causing them to rise.* Since damage to the eyes, nerves, and kidneys is similar in both Type I and Type II diabetes, the underlying cause is likely the same: high blood sugars.

Conventional Testing Not Enough

You may be thinking, "I test my blood sugars. I think I'm doing enough." Let's see what the DCCT found. At the start of the DCCT, the conventional group used urine testing and one or two injections a day. But by the end of the study 83 percent of this conventional group were testing their blood sugars and 91 percent were on two injections a day. Even with this improved therapy, their blood sugar control did not improve! In these people with diabetes who had volunteered for tight control at the start of the study, but were by chance assigned to the conventional care group, the mere testing of blood sugars had no effect on their control.

A major lesson from this study appears to be: *Learn as much as you can about your diabetes, and visit your specialized diabetes clinic regularly to get better blood sugars and have fewer complications.*

Eye and Kidney Disease

The DCCT showed that there is a direct relationship between a rise in blood sugar and the development of eye and kidney disease. The higher the rise in blood sugar, the greater the risk of these diseases. As blood sugar control worsens, there is a greater and greater risk for severe eye and kidney damage.

Heart Disease

Heart disease can happen to anyone, but heart attacks and strokes occur earlier, more often and with greater severity in those with diabetes. In the DCCT, 14 heart attacks occurred in the conventional control group, but only three heart attacks occurred in the intensive control group. This suggests that better blood sugars protect against heart attacks. However, the results are suggestive rather than conclusive because of the small number of heart attacks that occurred in the test groups.

How Complications Occur

Why do high blood sugars cause complications? To answer this, you need to know how damage occurs. Damage starts at the cell level. Cell health depends on a steady supply of fuel from glucose and free fatty acids. These fuels are regulated by insulin released directly into the blood from beta cells in the pancreas. If insulin levels are too low, too much glucose is released into the bloodstream by the liver. The result is a high blood sugar.

Cells in the eyes, kidneys, heart, blood vessels, and nervous system pick up glucose directly from the blood *without using insulin.* These cells are *more prone to damage from high blood sugars.* When blood sugars are high, cells in these organs are exposed to high internal levels of glucose.

The imbalance of sugar (glucose) means the cells are not receiving fuel the way they are meant to. Did you ever have water condensation in your gas tank? The sputtering in your car's engine that results from poor fuel is similar to the constant strain your cells undergo when blood sugars are too high.

These cells cannot perform normal functions well, if at all. Key enzymes are damaged and manufacture less of their products. Cells no longer repair themselves as normal cells do. The strain and breakdown over a period of time results in damage.

The importance of the high blood sugar environment to the development of complications is emphasized in studies of transplanted kidneys. When a kidney is taken from someone *without* diabetes and transplanted into someone *with* diabetes, kidney damage typical of diabetes often begins to develop in this nondiabetic kidney because of the high blood sugar environment into which it is placed.

A notable exception to this occurs when both a kidney and nondiabetic pancreas are transplanted together. Patients with dual transplants *who maintained normal blood sugars* were found to have no damage to their kidneys for periods as long as 10 years.

Some people escape serious health problems despite poor blood sugar control. Others will have only a single serious complication. Still others develop all the complications typical of diabetes, involving the eyes, kidneys, nerves and blood vessels.

Complications develop in people with high blood sugars. But other factors also determine whether and where damage will develop. These other factors include nutrition, exercise, blood pressure, smoking, alcohol intake, hormone levels, vitamin and mineral balance, and stress levels.

CAN COMPLICATIONS BE PREVENTED OR REPAIRED?

As we saw with the DCCT study, keeping blood sugars normal can definitely help prevent eye and kidney damage, circulation disorders and, possibly, heart problems. Prevention of cell damage starts with improved control of blood sugars.

Current research also suggests that damage can be slowed or stopped in all organs by improving control of blood sugars. And some damage appears to be reversible.

A study done in Oslo, Norway in the mid 1980s showed that people with Type I diabetes could repair nerve damage to some degree. A control group used conventional therapy of two shots a day. Another group used intensive therapy—an insulin pump or five or six injections a day. When this study tested nerve function, the intensive group (pump users in particular) showed no deterioration of nerve function at one year. They showed a slight improvement at two years. And they showed continuing nerve improvements over three and four years of better control.[2] Improved kidney function was also noted after four years.[3]

There are obvious limits to reversing damage. Cells like those in the eye and kidney can't be replaced or repaired once damage becomes severe. If a cell in the eye has been destroyed, vision cannot be restored to that area. If an eye cell is only partially damaged, however, indications are that the remarkable human body may be able to restore some of the lost function.

To arrest or repair complications through normal blood sugars, the treatment of diabetes faces major challenges. For example, many people with diabetes are not able to attain the excellent control achieved by subjects using the intensive therapies in studies like in the DCCT or others mentioned above. And despite the best interventions, a rollercoaster ride often takes blood sugars well above and below true normal.

Common sense tells us that the physical damage created in an environment of high blood sugars takes place over time and involves several mechanisms. Any improvement in blood sugar control lessens this damage. When blood sugars are normalized, some existing damage appears to be reversible.

How long might it take for good control to reverse damage? Interventions for kidney disease often show some immediate results, while repairing nerve damage takes much longer. The outlook for improvement as blood sugar control is normalized may be similar to that of a person who stops smoking. Once a smoker stops, it takes about seven years for the exsmoker's health risks to equal those of a nonsmoker. It is likely that a similar timetable for overcoming physical damage holds for those who improve their blood sugar control. How much damage can be reversed is unknown at this time.

SUMMARY

Blood sugar control is the most important way to prevent and repair damage. Other factors are also involved, but none is as important as the blood sugar. So the answer to "Why keep blood sugars normal?" is "To stay healthy and prevent or lessen complications."

Will an improved health picture be enough motivation to take on the challenge of blood sugar control? We hope so. Not only will your future health prognosis look rosier, but also you will start feeling better immediately when you get off the rollercoaster. The good feelings that come with stable and normal blood sugars are the important motivations for many.

The following chapters will provide the motivated reader with the tools to improve control, reduce blood sugar swings, and prevent long-term complications.

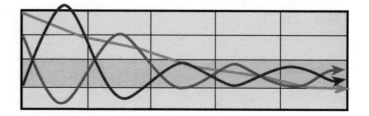

TYPES OF DIABETES AND HOW TREATMENT DIFFERS

2

There are several types of diabetes and each one has several stages of treatment. The stage of treatment a person is at depends to a great extent on how much residual insulin production he or she has. Someone who has no insulin production at all will benefit from more frequent injections of insulin, while someone with quite a bit of residual production may require only a single injection each day before their largest meal.

In this chapter we'll review:

- What diabetes is
- Different types of diabetes, their causes and symptoms
- How flexible insulin therapy is used with different types of diabetes

WHAT IS DIABETES?

About 16 million people in the U.S. have diabetes, which is actually several disorders that are grouped together because they all cause high blood sugars. Each form shares some defect related to insulin. When someone gets diabetes:

- Their beta cells are not making enough insulin, or,
- Due to the insulin resistance of other cells, the insulin does not do its job well.

Why is insulin essential to health? The body needs insulin to convert the food we eat into energy. Food is digested and broken down for use into many simpler substances. Two of these substances—glucose and fat—give us 90 percent of our energy. When insulin is absent or is not used well, glucose and fat will not provide normal amounts of energy.

In the healthy body, insulin is made and stored for use by beta cells in the pancreas, an organ that weighs about half a pound and sits behind the stomach. When insulin is released into the blood from the pancreas, it activates pathways on the outer walls of different cells so they can move glucose inside for use.

But if insulin is not made or not working well, glucose can't enter cells and it builds up instead in the blood. This sends blood sugars high, which is destructive to many of the body's systems. Furthermore, parts of the body become "starved" for fuel and, therefore, less healthy.

TYPES OF DIABETES

Diabetes is divided into two major types. People who have Type I diabetes depend on injected insulin to live because they produce little or no insulin themselves. This type, also called Insulin Dependent Diabetes Mellitus (IDDM), usually starts in children or young adults, but can happen at any age. In Type I diabetes, the insulin-producing beta cells are destroyed or severely damaged by an overactive immune system.

Type II diabetes, on the other hand, is called Non-Insulin Dependent Diabetes Mellitus (NIDDM) and usually starts when people are over 40. Type II is more likely to happen in those who carry excess weight around the middle. People with Type II diabetes produce insulin, but the insulin is not working well in the cells. Some 85 to 90 percent of all diabetes is Type II.

Both types of diabetes are quite treatable. Everyone with Type I diabetes needs to take insulin. Between 60 and 65 percent of those with Type II diabetes are able to achieve excellent control through modest weight loss, a healthier diet, regular exercise and the use of diabetes medications. The rest need to take injected insulin to control their blood sugar.

If either type of diabetes is left untreated or is treated poorly, very serious health problems may occur. If high blood sugars are not lowered, they may cause complications over time that can damage the eyes, kidneys and nerves. This can lead to blindness, kidney failure, or an amputation. Problems also often occur in fat and cholesterol metabolism that create a higher risk for heart and blood vessel disease. Good blood sugar control prevents this damage from happening. This prevention is a major goal of *Stop the Rollercoaster*.

Various studies are now underway to see if both types of diabetes can be prevented or cured. But in the meantime, treatment is very important. Keep in mind that paying attention to your diabetes every day has tremendous payoffs in your daily energy and health.

TYPE I DIABETES

Type I diabetes begins when the beta cells in the pancreas become severely damaged and are no longer able to make insulin. Insulin is the hormone that causes cells to produce glucose transporters and position them on the cell wall so that energy is created. Destruction of the beta cells is gradual and usually takes place over several years. When only 10 percent of the original beta cells remain, the blood sugar begins rising to dangerous levels. The person may feel fine up to this point, but will then rapidly develop symptoms typical of Type I diabetes.

These symptoms are fairly easy to identify because they are both unique and severe, and because they usually start in otherwise healthy children or young adults. The person becomes tired, very thirsty, and starts to urinate frequently during the day and night. Even though the person is eating more food, he or she loses weight.

Often, a very serious and life-threatening condition called ketoacidosis is underway when someone is first diagnosed with Type I diabetes. Since insulin is low, the blood sugar rises because the sugar is not being used as fuel in the cells. More fat is then released to replace the unusable sugar, making fat levels also rise.

Ketones, a by-product of fat metabolism, rise along with the fat levels. As the buildup of ketones in the blood progresses, the blood becomes more acidic and the person becomes quite ill. The person will suffer abdominal pain, become very dehydrated, and start to throw up. Immediate hospitalization may be required to save the person's life in this very dangerous situation. Ketoacidosis may also happen after the person has full-blown Type I diabetes if the blood sugars become very high because of an infection, illness, severe stress, or neglecting to take insulin.

Symptoms of Type I Diabetes
Excessive thirst
Frequent urination
Excessive tiredness
Irritability
Extreme hunger
Weight loss
Abdominal pain
Nausea
Fruity breath
Vomiting

What Causes Type I Diabetes?

Our immune system is designed to defend us against attack from foreign agents. It usually does not attack our own cells. But in Type I diabetes, an error occurs and the immune system begins attacking the beta cells by mistake. Destructive antibodies that are targeted against the beta cells can be measured in the blood long before the symptoms of Type I actually appear. It is now possible to measure these antibodies and identify who is likely to develop the disease.

Medical experts have not yet discovered exactly what triggers this change in the immune system. Genetics is important, but does not appear to be a dominant factor. When both parents have Type I diabetes, there is only a one in five chance that a child will get it. Also there seems to be little or no link to Type II diabetes. Some researchers believe that viruses or toxins in the environment trigger the immune system into its attack by changing the beta cells so they appear foreign to the body.

After this attack has destroyed the beta cells, the person's life depends on replacing natural insulin with injected insulin. Insulin is ideally given so that it mimics the pancreas' normal release of insulin. When insulin delivery is set up to mimic the pancreas, usually through the use of multiple injections or an insulin pump, Type I diabetes turns out to be a very manageable disease.

A person with Type I diabetes needs a long-acting background insulin through the day. Some background insulin *must always be present* in the blood to keep the blood sugar from rising while food is not being eaten. Then, a faster insulin is usually given before each meal to balance the food which is being eaten at that time. If insulin is delivered in this flexible way, blood sugars can be normalized. Add to this a healthy diet and regular exercise, and the person can look forward to a normal, healthy life.

Type II Diabetes

Type II diabetes, also called adult-onset diabetes and Non-Insulin Dependent Diabetes Mellitus (NIDDM), is more of a metabolic disorder. In Type II diabetes, the body does not use insulin well to control the blood sugar. In most cases of Type II diabetes, the beta cells in the pancreas are producing as much insulin as would be needed by someone else of equal weight. But changes in the cells which use insulin create resistance to insulin. As a result of insulin resistance, damaging high blood sugars occur.

About fifteen million Americans have Type II diabetes. Unfortunately, because of its gradual onset, half of the people who have it are unaware of their disease. By the time it is discovered, often 10 to 15 years of high blood sugars have passed.

Because of this common delay in diagnosis, serious complications may already be in progress at the time the disease is found. Therefore, a complete checkup for complications and associated diseases should be done as soon as the diabetes is discovered. Tests done at this time include a check of the blood pressure; a complete lipid panel for triglycerides, HDL, and total cholesterol; a microalbumin test of the urine to detect kidney changes; examination of the eyes by an ophthalmologist for retinopathy; examination of the feet for nerve and vascular problems; and a careful evelution of the heart.

Symptoms of Type II Diabetes
May be none
Weight gain
Tiredness
Irritability
Blurred vision
Numbness and tingling of feet
Frequent skin, bladder or vaginal infections
Slow healing

Symptoms of Type II diabetes start gradually and are often confused with normal aging. These symptoms include tiredness, frequent infections, irritability, blurred vision or changes in vision, and numbness and tingling in the feet and legs. Many people discover they have diabetes after a high blood sugar is found during a routine health exam.

Causes Of Type II Diabetes

The people most likely to develop Type II diabetes are people over 40 who have excess weight carried around the middle and who lead a sedentary lifestyle. People with a family history of Type II diabetes are more likely to get the disease, especially those from an Hispanic, Black or Native American background. The chances of developing Type II diabetes go up when a person has other signs of a relatively common disorder, called Syndrome X. This syndrome is found in one out of every four Americans. Signs of Syndrome X include insulin resistance, cholesterol problems (especially a low HDL and high triglycerides), high blood pressure, and a higher risk for heart disease.

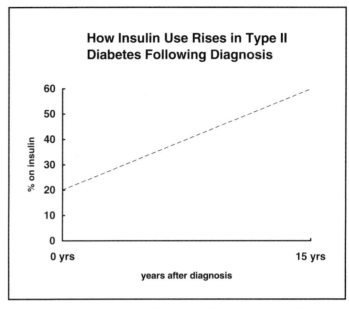

Fig. 2.1 Need For Insulin Over Time In Type II Diabetes

Eighty percent of those who develop Type II diabetes have a weight problem and some signs of Syndrome X. The insulin resistance that is present can best be treated through weight loss, a healthy diet, and exercise. Pills may also help in controlling blood sugars. If these approaches are not adequate, insulin may be needed. The other 20 percent of people with Type II diabetes are lean or normal weight and do not have insulin resistance. They often produce too little insulin and are likely to need insulin for blood sugar control. Altogether, 36 percent of those with Type II diabetes use insulin to aid with their control.

Treatment Of Type II

Keeping the blood sugars as normal as possible is the goal of treating Type II diabetes as well as Type I diabetes. People with this disease often do not feel bad when the blood sugar is 150, 200 or 250 mg/dl (8.3, 11.1, or 13.9 mmol), but damage is nevertheless taking place. As in Type I diabetes, this gradual damage can ultimately lead to blindness, amputation, kidney failure, impotence and other nerve problems.

Prevention of the problems found in Type II diabetes is easier than before with today's medications, and with day-to-day adjustments in nutrition, exercise, and stress management. The risk factors associated with this type of diabetes, like cholesterol and blood pressure changes, and even obesity, can be improved through proper use of medications. Several effective treatments are available for this form of diabetes.

For clarification, we like to break Type II diabetes into two groups. Knowing which subgroup of Type II diabetes you have assists you in treating it more effectively. We label these subgroups Type IIr and Type IIs:

Type IIr (or Type II with insulin *resistance*) In this most common form of diabetes, resistance to insulin in fat and muscle cells blocks the insulin's action. This resistance plus the loss of first-phase insulin release (insulin released in the first ten minutes after eating starts) creates rising blood sugars. Resistance to insulin is frequently found in people with an apple-shaped figure (excess weight around the middle). Resistance means that more insulin is needed to transport the same amount of glucose across cell membranes.

Cholesterol problems, high blood pressure, and heart disease are often associated with this resistance. Diet, exercise, oral agents, or insulin may be needed for control.

The Different Types of Diabetes

	Type I	Type IIr	Type IIs
Average age at onset	12	60	55
Typical age at onset	3-30	35-80	25-70
Percent of all diabetes	10 percent	75 percent	15 percent
Insulin problem	no insulin	resistance	too little insulin
Early treatment	i + d & e	p, + d & e	i or p, + d & e
Late treatment	i + d & e	i & p, + d & e	i + d & e

d = diet, i = insulin, p = pills, e = exercise

Table 2.2 Typical profiles of people with the three types of diabetes

Treatment here is focused on weight loss and on using exercise and medications to improve the action of insulin.

Type IIs (or Type II, but retaining *sensitivity* to insulin) Here the apple-shape is not present. In fact, the person may be slender, and sensitivity to insulin remains normal. Insulin production is gradually lost. Type IIs shares many features of Type I diabetes and may be a slow form of it. Here treatment focuses on improving insulin use with pills and on supplementing a reduced internal insulin production with injections of insulin.

Is Flexible Insulin Therapy For You?

If you have Type I diabetes, frequent, small doses of insulin are critical to achieving control. This means three or more injections a day. In our experience, well over 80 percent of those with Type I diabetes achieve better control and live a healthier life when they master flexible insulin therapy. In the early stages of Type IIs (sensitive) and Type IIr (resistant), a person's own internal insulin production may be quite adequate for good control and no insulin may be needed if adjustments are made in diet, exercise and weight. But as this internal production of insulin is lost over time, those with Type II diabetes are increasingly likely to benefit from insulin and flexible insulin therapy.

In early stages of Type II diabetes, only one injection may be necessary. With some internal production of insulin, one or two injections often provide excellent control for several years. As time passes, though, and as insulin production lessens, more frequent injections may be helpful. Anyone whose blood sugar control has not been satisfactory on one or two injections is likely to benefit from more frequent injections customized to their actual need.

Stages Of Therapy

Each type of diabetes has several stages of therapy. Although almost everyone with Type I diabetes goes straight to insulin, few people go straight to flexible insulin therapy. Below are the typical stages that a person with Type I diabetes passes through on their way to flexible insulin therapy with three or more injections, and an insulin pump if needed.

Typical stages for Type I diabetes are:

Stage One: Two injections of Regular plus a long-acting insulin before breakfast and dinner (This is minimum therapy in Type I diabetes. Only one injection a day is never recommended.)

Stage Two: Advance to flexible insulin therapy, with injections given three or more times a day

Stage Three: Use an insulin pump

The stages of therapy in Type II diabetes are more complicated than in Type I because there are more options: oral agents, diet, exercise and insulin. These stages are discussed in detail in Chapter 10.

WHEN DO YOU GO TO THE NEXT STAGE?

The decision to go to the next stage of therapy depends on how well the current treatment is working. Several factors, like the need for greater flexibility of meals and daily lifestyle, how stable your blood sugars are, and whether you are reaching your blood sugar and HbA_{1c} targets, all play a role.

There are two critical indicators that your current therapy is not effective. They give you the strongest reasons to advance to the next stage of therapy. Whenever the HbA_{1c} is staying more than 1 to 1½ percent above the upper limit for normal (for example, your lab's normal HbA_{1c} is 4.0 to 6.3 percent, but your readings have been 7.8 percent and higher), or the fasting and pre-meal blood sugars are often above 130 mg/dl (7.2 mmol).

Figure 2.3 gives help in interpreting your HbA_{1c} results. It shows your approximate average blood sugar revealed by your HbA_{1c} test. Each lab has a slightly different normal range, depending on the test they are using, but their normal values should be very close to 4% to 6%. Note the value for the intensive control group of the DCCT study. Try to keep your own HbA_{1c} near this value.

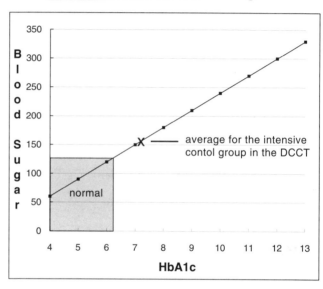

HbA1c Versus Blood Sugar

Figure 2.3 How to translate your HbA1c test into an average blood sugar through the day

Remember also that the blood sugars averaged here represent values *before and after* meals through an entire day, and not just the readings before meals!

Good judgement comes from experience;
and experience, well, that comes from bad judgement.

Anon.

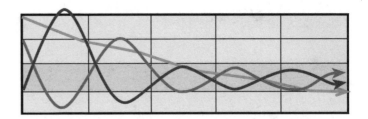

CAN FLEXIBLE INSULIN THERAPY HELP YOU?

3

Insulin is your most important tool in blood sugar control. It's what the body naturally uses for the job. But when the body's ability to create or to use insulin becomes damaged in diabetes, other approaches to control have to be found. Changes in diet, exercise, and diabetes medications work well for many people with Type II diabetes. But for everyone who has Type I and for the 36 percent of those with Type II diabetes who use insulin, the proper dosing and timing of injections becomes a major tool for control. In this book you can learn how to become a pro at using insulin to stop the highs and lows.

When doses of insulin are poorly matched to need, blood sugars vary. With the up-and-down swings in blood sugar come swings in emotion and energy. Even when the blood sugars show wide swings—43, 216, 51, 397, 36, 278 mg/dl—the person on the rollercoaster often doesn't realize how much this is affecting their personal life. Family members, however, are often quite concerned about these swings in the blood sugars, health and emotions.

Success in blood sugar control comes only when insulin is delivered in a way that mimics the normal pancreas. Because blood sugar control is so important to health, understanding how insulin therapy works and how to use it pays tremendous benefits. This book shows you how to match insulin doses to the needs in your own life.

What Is Flexible Insulin Therapy?

- Three or more injections a day, using Regular and an intermediate or long-acting insulin, or an insulin pump. (Many people with Type II diabetes continue producing much of their own insulin. Here, only one or two injections a day may be needed to achieve excellent control using flexible insulin therapy.)
- Four or more blood sugar tests each day
- A managed food intake through carb counting or other means
- Balancing events like exercise, menses and stress with adjustments in insulin and food
- Having defined targets—premeal and postmeal blood sugars, as well as the HbA_{1c}
- Staying aware of developments in diabetes
- Consulting your physician and other health personnel as needed
- Plus having more fun in your life because you're in control and feel better!

Table 3.1 FIT includes a variety of strategies to control blood sugars

FLEXIBLE INSULIN THERAPY

Flexible insulin therapy, or FIT, includes several elements (see Table 3.1 on the previous page). Other people call this approach "intensive control" or "multiple injections." We prefer the term flexible insulin therapy because it emphasizes the flexible lifestyle it allows. FIT uses multiple injections because they best imitate the normal pancreas. Insulin doses are changed as needed to match the changes that occur in a normal life. Experience has validated this flexible approach as the best way to improve the quality of life.

Another benefit of flexible insulin therapy, and the improved control that results, is the prevention of complications in the long run. Use of frequent injections for control has been widely promoted since the Diabetes Control and Complications Trial (DCCT) reported its results in June, 1993.[1] This major research study found people with Type I diabetes were healthier and developed far fewer complications when they controlled their blood sugars. Other research studies have found the same health benefits in Type II diabetes. Because of the findings of the DCCT, an advisory panel at the world famous Joslin Diabetes Center in Boston stated that *"three or more injections a day or use of an insulin pump should be recommended, unless clearly contraindicated."*[4]

Human nature being what it is, most people find that improvements in their day-to-day quality of life are a greater motivator than preventing long-range problems. People discover: "For the first time in years, I can eat when I want to," or I can really control my blood sugars now, and I feel better too."

People with Type I and Type II diabetes choose flexible insulin therapy for:
- A freer lifestyle
- More normal blood sugars
- Fewer and less severe insulin reactions
- The ability to vary the timing and size of meals
- Greater ability to exercise and maintain control
- Better control with travel or varied schedules
- Membership in a community of forward-thinking, health-conscious people
- Peace of mind

Physicians and health professionals recommend flexible insulin therapy for:
- Managing the Dawn Phenomenon
- Tight control during pregnancy
- Preventing, arresting or repairing complications
- Reducing wide blood sugar fluctuations in "brittle" diabetes
- Improving control during the growth spurts of adolescence
- Reducing insulin resistance in Type II diabetes

Stop the Rollercoaster shows how to reduce the ups and downs of metabolism and provides the tools to achieve excellent blood sugar control with appropriate insulin therapy.

ADVANTAGES OF FLEXIBLE INSULIN THERAPY

In addition to the benefits listed above, flexible insulin therapy appears to reduce by 35 to 75 percent the complications of diabetes, as demonstrated by the DCCT.

Good blood sugar control occurs when the body's need for insulin is matched with the amount of insulin delivered. There are two ways to do this. The first is to live a regulated lifestyle and take set doses of insulin to match this regulation. A more attractive alternative for many is to live a life with normal variety and learn to adjust daily insulin doses to match this variety. One diabetes specialist, Alan Marcus, M.D., summarized it this way: "A basic tenet of diabetes care is that the degree of lifestyle flexibility that can be achieved is directly related to the number of daily insulin injections." [5]

Under normal circumstances, the beta cells in the pancreas release precise amounts of insulin to cover two needs. First, the pancreas releases insulin into the blood around the clock, even when someone is not eating. This background insulin directs the release and use of glucose and, to some extent, fat as fuels. This background release of insulin can be mimicked by giving one or two doses each day of a long-acting insulin like Lente, NPH, or Ultralente in Type II diabetes, or with two or three doses of long-acting in Type I diabetes.

Second, under normal circumstances, short bursts of insulin are released by the pancreas into the blood to match the intake of carbohydrate from food. This larger, faster, meal-related release is mimicked by giving Regular or in the near future a new faster-acting insulin, called Lispro,® before meals. (Lispro is expected to be available in 1996.) Obviously, insulin delivery has to be both precise and flexible to meet these needs in an active lifestyle. This is where the advantage of flexible insulin therapy over conventional therapy with one or two injections a day really becomes apparent.

In diabetes, insulin is used to match three different needs:

First, insulin provides a relatively steady supply to match the background need. (Long-acting insulin covers this need.)

Second, insulin covers the carbohydrate in foods. (Carb Regular or Lispro insulin is used for this).

Third, insulin lowers high blood sugars to a normal range. (High Blood Sugar Regular or Lispro is used for this.)

MORE RELIABLE INSULIN ABSORPTION

Older approaches to insulin therapy often involved a single injection a day, for example an injection of 40 units of Lente before breakfast. With this injection, a large pool of long-acting insulin was placed under the skin to be absorbed over the next 24 to 36 hours.

Unfortunately, a large pool of insulin like this causes the blood sugar to vary. From day to day in the same individual, large variations in the amount of insulin actually absorbed from the injection site into the blood occur. The amount of long-acting insulin that actually reaches the blood from injection sites will vary by 25 percent, and range between 30 and 50 units, from one day to the next.[6] This variation becomes even more likely:

1. if the injection is placed near exercising muscles,

2. the skin is warmed by hot weather, or

3. the person takes a hot bath or sauna.

With short-acting insulins like Regular and Lispro, less variation occurs in day to day insulin absorption, usually 10 percent or less. A big advantage to multiple injections is that smaller amounts of long-acting insulin are used in each injection. Also, less insulin is used through the day.

For example, someone taking two injections a day might use 4 Regular and 28 Lente before breakfast and 5 Regular and 3 Lente before dinner. On switching to flexible insulin therapy, they might use three injections a day: 6 Regular and 18 Lente before breakfast, 5 Regular before lunch, and 7 Regular and 4 Lente before dinner. As this switch is made, the size of the morning long-acting insulin pool drops from 28 units on two injections a day to 18 units on three injections. Because less long-acting insulin is used, less variation occurs in insulin delivery.

MORE ACCURATE INSULIN DOSES

For convenience, many people use one or two injections a day instead of three or more. But this makes solving control problems difficult. If the blood sugar is high or low, it is harder to determine which insulin was poorly matched to need. "My blood sugar's high. I don't know if I covered dinner with too little Regular or if I need to raise my breakfast NPH," becomes a common dilemma.

With flexible insulin therapy, two injections of a long-acting insulin are used to minimize the rise and fall of the blood sugar when you are not eating. Then you take injections of Regular before each meal to cover carbohydrates in the food and, if needed, some extra Regular to reduce high blood sugars. Although this regimen may require three to five injections a day, each injection now has a specific purpose. In turn, this allows each insulin that is being injected to be individually tested and adjusted.

EASIER CONTROL

Some people believe they have been cursed with "brittle diabetes" because their blood sugars frequently rise and fall. People do vary in how easy it is for them to control their blood sugars. Those who are more sensitive to insulin are more likely to experience these blood sugar fluctuations. But "brittle diabetes" is most often caused by a poor match of insulin doses to lifestyle. Blood sugar fluctuation can largely be eliminated through better insulin dosing. (In some cases, living a steadier lifestyle does help. One teenager spotted his own part in his brittleness, "Why do I live wildly, when it just makes me feel bad?")

Control now becomes easier because each insulin's job is easy to understand. For instance, the long-acting insulin controls the blood sugar when no food is eaten. About 45 to 60 percent of the total daily insulin dose is delivered as long-acting insulin to do this job. This background insulin is first matched to background need to keep the blood sugar relatively stable while fasting. That's all the long-acting insulin does. It can be tested by not eating.

The rest of the daily insulin requirement is given as Regular:

- To cover the carbohydrate eaten in meals
- To lower unplanned high blood sugars to a normal range

Once the doses of long-acting insulin have been determined by testing, carbohydrates in different meals can be matched with a dose of Regular. This Carb Regular balances only the carbohydrate, measured in grams, through an easy method called carb counting. A blood sugar test taken four to five hours later will show if the dose of Carb Regular was correct for that meal. Because the long-acting insulin has already been tested and found to keep the blood sugar level when no eating occurs, any rise or fall beyond the expected range will show that the wrong amount of Regular was taken for that particular meal.

If the blood sugar goes high, an injection of High Blood Sugar Regular can be taken to bring the blood sugar down, based on the number of points (in mg/dl or mmol) the blood sugar drops per unit of Regular. If no food is eaten, a blood sugar taken four to five hours after this corrective dose should be close to normal. With flexible insulin therapy, insulin delivery is steadier and more predictable. This makes correction of high blood sugars safer. Because each insulin is doing its job, flexible insulin therapy makes blood sugars easier to control.

MORE VARIETY

People on flexible insulin therapy love the extra freedom. They express it like this: "I don't *have* to eat. I can wait till I feel hungry. This is the first time in years that I've actually felt hungry."

Another commented, "Just recently I began taking a more aggressive approach toward my diabetes, though diagnosed over 17 years ago when I was 10. After many failed attempts to monitor my blood sugars, I feel like I'm on the right track this time. I actually want to know what my blood sugars are. I started four shots a day months ago and love it. I have a new freedom."

Few people live rigid lives. Work hours vary, meetings and events pop up, meals are delayed or missed, and eating is often done on the run. On the weekends people rise early or sleep in late, exercise more or less and at different times of the day. Eating may involve large family meals or late dining after a movie.

With flexible insulin therapy, it's easy to eat meals late or to skip a meal entirely without the blood sugar falling. After the long-acting insulin is correctly set, a person may go all day with only an occasional snack and still maintain normal blood sugars. A person is no longer tied to waking up or eating at set times of the day, nor to having blood sugars bounce up and down as the demands of an active life are met.

BETTER CONTROL OF MORNING BLOOD SUGARS

Between 50 percent and 70 percent of those with either Type I or Type II diabetes find they need extra insulin in the early morning hours to offset a rise in their blood sugar.[7] Called the Dawn Phenomenon for obvious reasons, this sugar rise in Type I diabetes is triggered by a normal daily increase in growth hormone production during the early morning hours. Growth hormone causes the liver to produce and release more sugar.

In Type II diabetes, a similar rise is triggered by insulin resistance and excess abdominal weight. When someone stops eating during the night, fatty acids from fat stores in the abdomen start to be released into the blood. The greater the excess fat in the middle, the more likely the blood sugar rise becomes. The release of excess fat is often seen as high triglyceride levels. Some fats cause resistance to insulin. The liver interprets this excess fat and relative "lack of insulin" as a low blood sugar and starts making glucose. Meanwhile, the muscle cells which have also become resistant to insulin cannot use as much of the excess glucose produced by the liver, and the blood sugar rises overnight.

Whatever the cause, if the extra glucose produced is not offset by a rise in the insulin level, the blood sugar will rise as dawn approaches. Taking more long-acting insulin at dinner or bedtime balances the excess glucose being produced by the liver and helps the muscles pick up more glucose from the blood.

> ### Tip For Type II
>
> In Type II diabetes, loss of excess abdominal weight is the best solution for correcting high morning blood sugars and high sugars in general. But a trick that John Walsh uses with his patients to blunt this overnight rise is to have them eat a complex carbohydrate, like a green apple, at bedtime. The slow release of carbohydrate from digestion of the green apple lessens the amount of fat released during the night and in many people lowers the morning reading!

Why is this important? Because the first blood sugar of the day is the *most important one for controlling the entire day's readings.* When high, it is often difficult to bring down because the liver's production of glucose is hard to turn off after it starts. To compound the problem, lowering the high reading with extra Regular at breakfast and again at lunch makes an afternoon insulin reaction likely. "If I wake up high, my whole day is shot!" is a typical complaint.

Evening Injections

With a Dawn Phenomenon, the liver begins creating and releasing extra glucose into the blood at around 3 or 4 a.m. To prevent this, a precisely-timed increase in insulin is needed at 1 or 2 a.m. The type and dose of the evening long-acting insulin can be adjusted to keep the blood sugar from rising. So multiple injections can be used to deliver insulin correctly during the night. "I now wake up in the morning with a normal blood sugar!" is a common joy for people after they have fine-tuned their insulin to this need.

Occasionally someone with a strong Dawn Phenomenon finds it difficult to match this early morning insulin need with *any* injected insulin regimen. But, as detailed in later chapters, *Stop the Rollercoaster* will give you your best shot (pun intended) at controlling the morning reading. However, a small fraction (probably three percent to 10 percent of those with Type I diabetes) will continue to find it difficult to control their morning reading with injections. In this more difficult group, control can usually be regained with an insulin pump.

REDUCED INSULIN DOSES

Many people are on too much insulin. When blood sugars are brought under good control, total doses tend to be reduced. If insulin reactions are being caused by too much insulin, their severity and frequency will be lessened as less insulin is used.

Reactions occur *frequently* if insulin doses are slightly too high through the day. They become *severe* when the insulin level is much too high at one time of the day.

Reactions happen:

- When too much insulin has been injected
- When insulin is taken but a meal is miscalculated, missed, or delayed
- When the amount or timing of long-acting insulin is misjudged
- When insulin under the skin is absorbed more quickly than usual, such as when exercise or heat increases blood flow

Fear of insulin reactions is a common reason people avoid intensive control. They feel that attempting to lower high blood sugars may lead to lows.

Here again, the advantage of frequent injections can be seen. Small doses of Regular insulin given frequently are ideal for those whose mealtimes are irregular and those who are sensitive to insulin. Taking several, smaller injections of insulin in a planned way allows someone to lower highs while avoiding lows because insulin doses are better matched to need.

Another benefit noted by some people using flexible insulin therapy is that when an insulin reaction occurs, it is less severe. As insulin delivery matches need more closely, the blood sugar drops more slowly and gives extra time in which to recognize the symptoms of a low blood sugar. As reaction time lengthens, it's easier to remedy the situation before it becomes severe.

FEWER COMPLICATIONS

Fuzzy vision? Albumin leaking into the urine? You'll notice the change in vision, but you will not be aware of excess albumin in your urine unless a special microalbumin test is done. Such signs of beginning complications related to diabetes are another reason to consider better control.

Can flexible insulin therapy help if you already have complications? Yes, in many cases! When you better understand how insulin works, you can more easily control your blood sugar. This control helps cells and organs to become healthier. Having a better handle on blood sugar control, in turn, increases motivation and inspires a healthier lifestyle. See Chapter 29 for more information on this.

ADVANTAGES FOR TYPE II DIABETES

People with Type ll diabetes can also benefit from flexible insulin therapy. You may think frequent injections are only for those with Type I diabetes. But flexible insulin therapy offers these advantages for those with Type IIr diabetes:

- Blood sugar control can be achieved with *less insulin*.[8, 9] Blood insulin levels are lower and the improved blood sugar control improves the sensitivity to insulin. Most diabetes specialists believe this translates directly into better health, as has already been shown in Type I diabetes with the DCCT Study.

- *Weight loss* is easier because meal carbohydrates and calories can be lowered at any time by lowering the Carb Regular at the same time. Also, there is less need to overeat to compensate for low blood sugars due to excess insulin.

- There is less overproduction of insulin and *less strain* on the beta cells that make insulin.

- *Triglyceride levels* are lowered. Triglyceride levels are often dangerously high in Type II diabetes. These levels often rise along with the blood sugars and are a risk factor for heart disease.

Flexible insulin therapy can also help those with Type IIs which develops in thin, older people. These individuals are sensitive to insulin and often benefit from using smaller doses of insulin given more frequently.

ADVANTAGES OVER INSULIN PUMPS

Flexible insulin therapy shares many of the advantages offered by an insulin pump. Pumps have an advantage in how precisely insulin can be delivered, but in a couple of other areas, FIT has the advantage.

Lower Costs

In 1994 dollars, the cost for syringes ranged from $36 (reuse of syringes) to $291 a year (single use) for someone taking four injections a day. Compare these figures to supplies for a pump which range from $362 to $1,342 a year, plus an additional $900 a year averaged over five years ($4,500 total) to cover the cost of the pump itself.[10] There are obvious cost advantages to multiple injections.

Less Risk Of Ketoacidosis

When a long-acting insulin is injected under the skin, this subcutaneous pool continues to release insulin over the next 24 hours with NPH or Lente insulins, and over the next 30 hours with Ultralente insulin. On a pump, only a small pool of Regular insulin is present under the skin. If insulin delivery from a pump is interrupted, blood sugars can start to rise in 90 minutes or less. Three hours after insulin delivery is interrupted, the level of insulin in the blood may drop to only 60 percent of its starting level. This is when the person on the pump is vulnerable to ketoacidosis.

As insulin levels drop, cells stop using glucose as fuel and begin to rely on fat as fuel. More and more fat is burned. This causes an excessive buildup of by-products called ketones in the blood. A dangerous acidic state, called ketoacidosis, develops. In studies done on insulin pumps in the early 1980s, ketoacidosis requiring an emergency room or hospital visit happened on average once in every six and a half years of pump use.[11] Although pump therapy has undergone major advances which have decreased the risk, ketoacidosis still occurs once for every 16 to 18 years of pump use and remains more likely on a pump than with injections.[12]

Skin Problems

Skin irritation and rashes are common on pumps. An infection at the infusion site is also more likely than at an injection site. These problems don't occur with injections.

Drawbacks Of Flexible Insulin Therapy

Inconvenience

Giving smaller injections of insulin through the day requires that a syringe, insulin, and blood testing equipment be available. As armies quickly discover, wars are won largely by the availability of supplies. Blood sugar control is no different, and the tools used to win the health war have to be available. You have to fill prescriptions and keep needed supplies at home, in the office and in your car. You must also make time to administer frequent injections and tests in spite of other demands that may arise.

Someone on flexible insulin therapy has to be committed to testing and injecting before meals and at any point of the day. Supplies cannot be left at home or forgotten. Despite the obvious health benefits, some people will choose not to follow a FIT regimen.

Fear Of Embarrassment

Some people are not ready to face exposing their diabetes through frequent testing and use of multiple daily injections. This is especially true if they feel other people will perceive them as being different or as having a "disease." The teen years and early twenties are particularly difficult ages to be perceived as different. The stigma of taking a shot before each meal may make its use impractical for some at these ages. To some it may seem inconvenient, annoying or embarrassing.

After beginning flexible insulin therapy, however, most people are surprised at how easy it is. The feared personal rejection and inconvenience become instead the respect of friends and relatives as they notice that blood sugars and emotions are better controlled.

Increased Risk Of Insulin Reactions

The Diabetes Control and Complications Trial (DCCT) clearly showed that the major drawback in attempting to improve blood sugar control was an increased risk of insulin reactions. As you attempt to control blood sugars, you will most likely have lower target blood sugars than before. Severe insulin reactions, requiring the assistance of another person, were three times as likely in the intensive control group, and occurred whether multiple injections or an insulin pump were being used.[1] Some participants had several episodes and others had none at all.

An episode of severe hypoglycemia occurred every year and a half on average in the intensive group, compared to only once every five years in the control group.[1] Episodes of unconsciousness or seizure due to low blood sugar occurred once every six years in the intensive group compared to once every 20 years in the control group. However, the overall benefit of lower risks for eye, kidney, and nerve damage were judged to outweigh the increased risk for hypoglycemia.

Anyone wanting to improve their control has to be aware of this extra risk. However, planning, monitoring, attention, and information can greatly reduce this risk.

Hypoglycemia Unawareness

When someone has a low blood sugar but doesn't recognize it, the condition is called hypoglycemia unawareness. Someone other than the person with diabetes recognizes the low sugar symptoms. Hypoglycemia unawareness can be dangerous, especially when the person who has it is convinced he or she doesn't have it and refuses to treat it. This condition happens more often when someone has had diabetes for a number of years, when a meal is skipped for which insulin was taken, when insulin doses are excessive, with abuse of alcohol, or after extra activity.

These severe insulin reactions become more likely as blood sugars overall are brought closer to normal. The reason for this is that insulin reaction symptoms are harder to feel when blood sugars drop more gradually, and as more time is spent near the hypoglycemic range. This is also true when a person's normal warning signals become weaker due to frequent lows.

On the other hand, if flexible insulin therapy is used well it can actually *reduce* the risk of hypoglycemia unawareness. As smaller insulin doses are delivered dependably and physiologically, and attention is paid to matching insulin doses to normal changes in lifestyle, severe hypoglycemia becomes less likely. Also, there is more time to recognize that a reaction is underway.

Changes In Retinopathy

Some people who improve their control rapidly with an insulin pump have been found to experience a *temporary worsening* of existing eye damage. Researchers believe this unexpected damage may be caused by a rise in insulin-like growth factors or by the sudden lowering of previously excessive glucose supplies. This worsening of existing eye damage has been documented when blood sugars are rapidly improved with an insulin pump.[13,14] It may also occur when control is suddenly improved with injections.

If your blood sugar control has not been great and you have retinopathy (damage to the eye's retina), your physician may advise that you improve your control gradually. With existing retinopathy, you want to be followed by an experienced ophthalmologist as you begin improving blood sugars. This monitoring ensures that the eye damage does not get worse during this period. If eye changes do worsen, it is likely to be temporary and should improve after the first few months of control. But see your ophthalmologist to verify this.

SUMMARY

Flexible insulin therapy has distinct advantages in the control of blood sugars. Compared to older therapies, it offers consistent insulin delivery and comes closer to maintaining normal blood sugars. This therapy allows high blood sugars to be rapidly and safely corrected. With improved blood sugars, the risk of developing health problems related to diabetes lessens. Several research studies have also documented some repair of existing complications.

Flexible insulin therapy allows for a more normal daily life: the ability to skip meals, eat late, and cover variations in carbohydrate intake. Quick adjustments can be made when high blood sugars, exercise, or illnesses occur.

By more closely mimicking the function of the normal pancreas, the extra injections allow freedom. This may seem like a frivolous reason for taking extra injections to someone who does not have diabetes. But to someone who has had to eat meals on a rigid schedule, who must have a carbohydrate snack every night before bed, who occasionally wakes up in a soaking sweat at 3 a.m., who faces high blood sugars every morning, who suffers from lows when exercising, who cannot eat spontaneously, who has returned to consciousness in an emergency room with an intravenous catheter in the arm, or who simply wants to sleep late on the weekend, flexible insulin therapy is a pleasure.

A little inconvenience is more than offset by the improved sense of well-being and a more flexible lifestyle. For many people, flexible insulin therapy offers clear advantages in the quest for a healthy lifestyle with normal blood sugars. To see how you might benefit from flexible insulin therapy, take the self-test (Table 3.2) on the next page.

ARE YOU A GOOD CANDIDATE FOR FIT?

How well does your current program work? To find out, circle the number on each question below that best describes you. Total up your score and compare it to the scorecard to see how close you are to achieving flexible insulin therapy:

The FIT Scale

1. How motivated are you to control your own blood sugars?

   not very   0   1   2   3   4   5   very   _____

2. Number of blood sugar tests you do each day:

            0   1   2   3   4   5   6 (or more)   _____

3. Number of injections/day?

            0   1   2   3   4   5   6 (pump = 6)   _____

4. Do you record your test results?

            yes   (5 pts)   no   (0 pts)   _____

5. Do you use your blood sugar tests to adjust your insulin?*

            yes   (5 pts)   no   (0 pts)   _____

6. Do you adjust your Regular to individual meals by carb counting or other means?*

            yes   (5 pts)   no   (0 pts)   _____

7. Do you adjust your Regular to lower high blood sugars?*

            yes   (5 pts)   no   (0 pts)   _____

8. Do you adjust L, NPH, or UL to meet varying needs, such as exercise or illness?*

            yes   (5 pts)   no   (0 pts)   _____

9. Do you get a regular lab test to evaluate your control (a HbA_{1c} or fructosamine test at least every 6 mos.)?

            yes   (5 pts)   no   (0 pts)   _____

10. Do you call your physician when control problems occur?

            yes   (5 pts)   no   (0 pts)   _____

                           Total   =   _____

* Seek your physician's help on insulin adjustments until he or she is confident that you can make your own adjustments.

Flexible Insulin Therapy Scorecard

Score:	What it means:
0-9	Who is really in control here?
10-19	Honesty pays! Where to improve?
20-29	Close. Where can you improve?
30-39	Terrific! Minor improvements.
40-50	Wow! You're there.

Table 3.2   A self-test to evaluate your current care versus FIT

THE FLEXIBLE INSULIN THERAPY CHECKLIST

The FIT Checklist guides you to chapters in the book where you can find the help you need. Answer "Yes" to each question before proceeding. If you answer "No", correct your control at that step.

For example, if your long-acting insulin has not been correctly set, it won't be possible to set your doses of Carb Regular until this has been done.

✓ The Overnight Long-Acting Insulin

Can you go to bed with a blood sugar of 80 to 120, eat little or no snack and wake up in the morning with a normal reading?   **No** ▶ Review Chapters 13 & 14

Yes ▼

✓ The Daytime Long-Acting Insulin

With a normal blood sugar before a meal, can you skip that meal (no Carb Reg., of course), and have your blood sugar stay level or fall no more than 30 points over the next 4 to 5 hours?   **No** ▶ Review Chapters 13 & 14

Yes ▼

✓ Your Carb Counting

Can you determine the grams of carbohydrate in foods you are eating, either through carb counting, food exchanges or by using another dietary system?   **No** ▶ Review Chapter 8

Yes ▼

✓ The Carb Regular

With a normal blood sugar before a meal, can you cover the carbohydrate in the meal with Regular so that your blood sugar is normal 4 to 5 hours later?   **No** ▶ Review Chapters 13 & 15

Yes ▼

✓ High Blood Sugar Regular

When you have a high blood sugar, can you take a dose of Regular so that your blood sugar is normal 4 to 5 hours later?   **No** ▶ Review Chapters 13 & 16

Yes ▼

✓ For Overlapping Regular

In situations where you use 2 or more injections of Regular in a short period of time, can you give these injections without causing an insulin reaction?   **No** ▶ Review Chapter 17

Yes ▼

✓ Your Handling Of Reactions

When you have a low blood sugar, are you able to recognize and handle it by yourself, and keep your blood sugar from bouncing above 150 mg/dl afterward?   **No** ▶ Review Chapters 19 & 20

Yes ▼

✓ Your Handling Of Exercise

When you exercise, can you avoid severe reactions and keep your blood sugar between 70 and 150 mg/dl (3.9 to 8.3 mmol)?   **No** ▶ Review Chapters 21 & 22

Yes ▼

Terrific! Check again later!

TAKING CONTROL

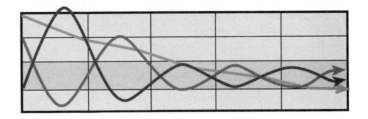

DIABETES AND THE HEALTH CARE SYSTEM

4

Managing your health with diabetes involves learning about the health care system and the standards of care related to your personal program of therapy. It's also wise to keep current on the latest research developments in the treatment and prevention of problems common in diabetes.

In addition, you will want to get the best results possible from the considerable financial investments you are making.

This chapter will cover how to:

- Evaluate your current health care system
- Take more responsibility for your own health
- Learn what you can do to prevent common complications of diabetes
- Work to improve your health care system

HOW GOOD IS YOUR HEALTH CARE?

Do you have your eyes examined each year by an opthalmologist to reduce risk of eye damage? Is your HbA_{1c} tested every three months to monitor your blood sugar levels? Does your doctor administer a yearly urine microalbumin test to detect early kidney disease?

If you answered no to any of the above, you will want to read this chapter carefully. The Diabetes Control and Complications Study set a new "Standard of Care" for Type I diabetes that should be followed by every health care practitioner working with every person with Type I unless there are clear reasons not to do so. This new standard sets the guidelines by which health practitioners evaluate their patients and advise and train them to care for themselves. This standard, with minor adjustments for age, is just as appropriate for people with Type II diabetes.

Table 4.1 shows the minimum recommendations for an effective health care program that both maintains optimum health and reduces risks of complications.

How Health Care Profits Affect Your Treatment

If the new Standard of Care is recognized as the best way to manage diabetes, can every person with diabetes expect to receive the training, testing, and support it recommends? Does your health care system act as if an ounce of prevention is worth a pound of cure? The answer from too many heath care delivery systems these days is, "Not necessarily."

For better or worse, medical care today often sets policy and makes decisions based on profit and the bottom line. Cost containment has become a major goal in medicine. This policy often means that more patients are seen by fewer health care practitioners for shorter segments of time. "Get 'em in, provide minimal service, and get 'em out," has become the underlying theme in too many health care settings.

Poor Delivery of Medical Services

In diabetes, less frequent and shorter clinic visits translate into poorer long-term health. The medical care given by one large HMO was analyzed by researchers at Cedar-Sinai Research Institute in Los Angeles. The care that was being delivered was found to be far below minimum standards. Over a one year period (1993), only four percent of this HMO's clients with diabetes had their eyes checked by an ophthalmologist (a physician who specializes in eye care).

Only six percent received a foot exam, and only 44 percent had their HbA_{1c} tested. The HbA_{1c} results in over a third of these people were higher than the values in the conventional ("poor") care group of the DCCT where so much damage occurred. Only one in twenty saw an endocrinologist, one in ten saw a dietician, and one in twelve attended a class in diabetes at any time during that year.

Mayer Davidson, M.D., an internationally recognized authority in diabetes and a researcher involved in this study, summarized the study in an understated way: "Diabetes care provided in HMOs does not meet the ADA Standard of Care and may not provide adequate follow-up to help patients with diabetes avoid the development of long term complications."[15]

TAKING CARE OF YOURSELF

"What, if anything, can I do about all this?" might be the question you are asking yourself about

Standard Of Care Recommendations
• Keep blood sugars as close to normal as possible.
• Monitor blood sugars at home in everyone with Type I diabetes and everyone with Type II diabetes who has erratic readings or an elevated HbA_{1c}.
• Inject three or more times per day or use an insulin pump in Type I and Type II diabetes when blood sugar control is not adequate with fewer injections.
• Record blood sugars and use the results to adjust insulin doses, foods eaten, and exercise to maximize blood sugar control.
• Do an HbA_{1c} (or fructosamine) test every 3 months to monitor the level of control.
• Educate everyone with diabetes about self care.
• Do a yearly urine microalbumin test to detect kidney disease at an early stage, and reduce the need for dialysis or transplant.
• Do a yearly total lipid panel to measure cholesterol, triglycerides and HDL ("protective cholesterol"), and overall risks for heart disease.
• Get a yearly eye exam to detect eye damage and prevent vision loss.

Table 4.1: Does your health care measure up?

now. The best answer is to be aware of the situation and to take as much responsibility as possible for managing your own day-to-day health care. Taking care of diabetes is always best done by a knowledgeable, highly motivated individual who sees himself or herself as involved, responsible, empowered, and as an important member of the health care team.

Good health care requires that you commit yourself to learning about diabetes. (Reading this book is a great start!) Prioritize your goals to better mange diabetes in your life. Identify the questions you have about your own health care. Keep asking these questions until you get answers you can understand and *act upon*.

Fortunately, physicians and other health care providers prefer to work with people who are interested in promoting their own health. A good health provider loves people who ask questions, who want to learn, and who take responsibility for living healthier lives. Why is this?

It's easier to solve problems when two minds are working together and greatly improves the chances for a positive outcome. Health care providers love success. They respect an involved, responsible person. They love working with someone who watches their diet, exercises regularly, tests and records their blood sugars and learns how to use this feedback to improve their control.

Put Yourself in Your Doctor's Shoes

Think about diabetes for a moment from the other side. The following four scenarios describe different approaches you can take toward keeping records that help your doctor assist you in controlling your blood sugars. Put yourself into each scenario as you read it:

Scenario One: You walk into your doctor's office for a checkup. When he/she asks if you've been testing your blood sugars, you say: "I left my records at home, but I always check my blood sugars and they're OK." Your doctor responds, "Great, keep up the good work!" Meanwhile he/she is thinking "Sure, this is the 19th time I've heard that this week. Probably doesn't record or care. I'll have to do a HbA_{1c} to find the truth and hope they come back for the next visit."

Scenario Two: Same situation, but this time you say, "I don't write my readings down, but I brought my meter. It's got a memory." Your physician answers, "Great, let's take a look," thinking "At least they're testing. Too bad there's no way to figure out why the blood sugar is doing whatever it's doing from the meter's memory. I don't have time to write out their record. Let's look at three or four readings, and get the HbA_{1c} test to see how bad the situation really is."

Scenario Three: Same situation, but this time you've also brought sheets of paper that contain your blood sugar readings over the last month. Your doctor smiles, and after looking at the record, says "Looks like you're having low blood sugars in the afternoon two or three times a week. Some of them look quite low. You must feel pretty bad when these hit. Why is your blood sugar dropping so low only on *some* days? Are you exercising on those days, or is it what you're eating at lunch?" You realize you don't really know why this is happening.

"Well, that's splendid, Mrs. Johnson. I'm so pleased you have at least considered thinking about the remote possibility that you may sometime in the future actually have a notion to purchase a blood glucose meter to help you monitor this pesky little diabetes problem..."

Scenario Four: Same situation, but this time you walk into your doctor's office with comprehensive records. Each chart shows one day's results with blood sugars graphed out, the grams of carbohydrate in each food, insulin doses, the duration and intensity of your exercise, and comments about foods or unusual stress that seem to affect your readings. Your doctor intently looks over your records and says, "Looks like those afternoon lows always happen when you play golf in the morning and eat pasta for lunch. You might need less Regular for those pasta lunches, or maybe a dessert with an extra 30 to 40 grams of carbohydrate. What do you think?"

"Your blood pressure's great. Your last HbA_{1c} and triglyceride levels were both normal. By the way, have you seen the ExCarb system that shows how many grams of carbohydrate it takes to balance different activities? And have you thought about joining that new research study on exercise and diabetes over at the university?" Meanwhile, your doctor is thinking, "Wow, these records are great! I wish everyone took this much responsibility for their health."

Keep Good Records

These scenarios dramatize the difference your records can make in your health care. Helping your health care provider makes sense. Studies show that recording blood sugars on paper brings the readings down. And health providers spend more time during clinic visits with people who bring good diabetes records with them.

Are all records equal? We hope these scenarios have convinced you they are not. But what does a "great record" mean? Health providers are not magicians. They can't look at the raw data from a meter or logbook and know why your blood sugars are going high or low. Most of these simple recording devices don't record how many carbs and calories you're eating, or what your activity and stress levels are. Only recently have a few advanced meters begun to incorporate data collection systems that allow the user to record food or carbohydrate intake, insulin doses, activity and exercise levels, and even stress.

Find Your Blood Sugar Patterns

If you're using a simple logbook, you hand your physician a list of your blood sugar readings. For some with Type II diabetes whose blood sugars do not vary greatly, a simple logbook may be sufficient. But for many, these logbooks do not give enough information to identify and correct problem areas in control. No patterns, no meaningful analysis, no conclusions about solutions. A logbook called the Blood Sugar Inventory, presented in the next chapter, takes the logbook concept a step further.

The ideal way to address control problems is to have your data displayed graphically. A chart reveals patterns of high and low blood sugars, along with their relationship to insulin doses, food intake, exercise, and stress. Some advanced record books, like the Smart Charts in Chapter 6, allow information affecting the blood sugars to be displayed in a graphic format. Each one-day chart provides space for data to be recorded and displayed in a way that reveals at a glance the reasons for up and down patterns. Use of Smart Charts is covered in Chapter 6.

Look at the records in Figure 4.2 below and see for yourself whether a simple logbook or a charting system tells you more, and better helps you take action.

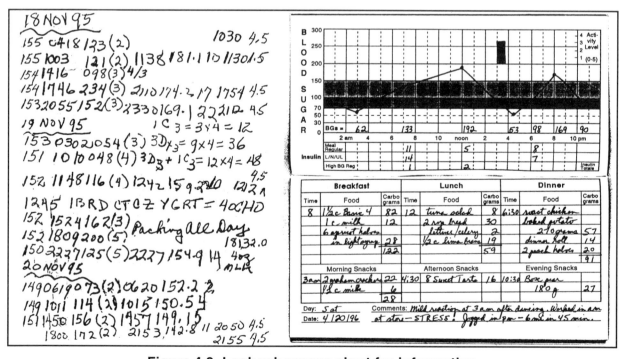

Figure 4.2 Logbook versus chart for information

AN ENTHUSIASTIC PHYSICIAN IS GOOD MEDICINE

To weave your way through the medical system, receive appropriate medical care, and have meaningful feedback on the records you bring in, the best advice we can give is to have an enthusiastic physician working with you. Correct treatment of diabetes requires a very specialized understanding of this disease. This care is best provided by a physician whose practice is focused on diabetes. When your physician or other health care provider has a positive attitude and encourages you to care for yourself, your path to good health becomes easier.

Learn About Your Health Care Team

Know the people who treat you. What is their experience? Have they taken extra specialty training in diabetes? How many of their patients have diabetes? What is their reputation in the community for diabetes care? Will they refer you to specialists like a retina specialist or dietician when appropriate?

Will they order appropriate lab tests? Do they do a complete physical, and check your blood pressure and feet regularly? Do they discuss their findings with you? These are the issues that let you know if you are receiving good diabetes care. Many of the solutions in day-to-day issues in blood sugar management can be provided by qualified subspecialists like certified diabetes educators (C.D.E.) and dieticians. Know your whole health care team.

Set Your Own Goals

As management consultant Steven Covey says, "*Always begin with the end in mind.*" Take some time to consider the changes you'd like to make in your life with diabetes.

To clarify your goals, circle the number in Figure 4.3 that describes the importance of each goal. Place goals that are important to you more clearly into focus and you will be able to more easily achieve them.

How important are these goals to you?	not very				very
A freer lifestyle	1	2	3	4	5
Feeling better	1	2	3	4	5
A lower HbA$_{1c}$ (fructosamine)	1	2	3	4	5
Fewer reactions	1	2	3	4	5
Stop/reverse complications	1	2	3	4	5
A healthy, long life	1	2	3	4	5
A healthy pregnancy	1	2	3	4	5
Other_____	1	2	3	4	5

Figure 4.3 Targeting your goals is the first step to achieving them.

FINANCIAL STRAIN OF DIABETES

A person's yearly costs for four daily blood sugar tests with a meter and four injections a day average between $925 and $1,175 a year.[16] As costly as supplies are, this is far from the worst of it. When poor control progresses into complications involving the kidneys, heart or eyes, costs really escalate. End Stage Renal Disease (ESRD), which requires dialysis or kidney transplantation now costs close to $10 billion a year, averaging $45,000 a year for each person who needs dialysis or a transplant.[17] Diabetes is currently the leading cause of kidney failure and blindness in this country. Laser treatment, blindness and amputations are expensive in both financial and emotional terms. Diabetes ends up costing 11.9 percent of *all the money* spent on medical care in the United States, some $92 billion a year in 1992 dollars.[18]

THE LONGTERM GOAL OF PREVENTING DIABETES

From a strictly economic point of view, the medical costs of diabetes and its associated complications, as indicated in the previous paragraph, mandate preventive health measures. The goal can be reached through two paths. First is the early detection of complications in the person with diabetes. Most health damage can be prevented if detected early. The Standard of Care in Table 4.1 provide guidelines to prevent complications. The second step is prevention of diabetes itself. Researchers are actively pursuing the prevention of both Type I and Type II diabetes.

Prevention Of Type I Diabetes

Causes for Type I diabetes are beginning to be understood, but identifying all of those who are at risk appears unlikely. A large study is underway in the United States to test the first degree relatives (children, brothers and sisters, and parents) of a person who already has Type I diabetes.

Unfortunately, this study will identify only a fraction of those at risk. Some 70 percent of people who develop Type I diabetes have no close relative with the disease, so they would not be screened in this way. A comprehensive screening program would require that specialized lab tests be done for all children in the U.S. every two to four years. Costs to do this screening would likely be higher than the lifetime economic costs of the disease itself.

A more economical intervention might be available, though. Nicotinamide, an inexpensive relative of the B vitamin niacin, was found as early as 1950 to protect animals against Type I diabetes.[19] More recent clinical trials aimed at the prevention of Type I diabetes with nicotinamide have been promising. A much larger clinical trial, called ENDIT, based largely in Europe, is now underway to test this approach.

Prevention Of Type II Diabetes

Type II diabetes presents a different problem. Although it's easier to identify people who are at risk of Type II diabetes because it is more clearly inherited, this disease is increasing at epidemic rates as the population ages, and as the world's lifestyles and diets become more westernized. Type II diabetes is largely a consequence of reduced physical activity combined with weight gain, especially when this weight is added around the middle.

Lifestyle changes (a low fat, low calorie diet, plus daily exercise) would prevent much of Type II, but these changes are overwhelmingly difficult to implement, as demonstrated by the alarming failure of weight loss programs.

NEED FOR A NEW PUBLIC HEALTH POLICY

Unfortunately, the long-term view needed to carry out preventive health care is often blinded by the search for short-term profits. The financial horizon on which health care decisions are made stretches no further than 12 to 24 months. Preventive measures that pay dividends in 5, 10 or 15 years have little chance for support. Chronic diseases like diabetes that will be with the person for a lifetime do not fare well in today's shortsighted medical environment.

Here are some suggestions for legislative solutions:

• A mandate against discrimination. No applicant can be turned down by any health insurance system for any preexisting health problem, nor dropped if a health problem appears. This is especially important with diabetes because studies show that people who have diabetes cost a health care system three and a half times as much as the average.

• Special attention should be paid to policies that create medical irresponsibility. For instance, 72 percent of the costs of End Stage Renal Disease (ESRD) in people with diabetes are paid by Medicare (and all of us). Swedish researchers have reported that ESRD rates in Type I diabetes in Sweden have already fallen from 30 percent to 10 percent due to improved blood sugar control.[20]

Kidney disease in diabetes can obviously be prevented and its progression greatly slowed. But insurers have less incentive to do these interventions as long as they can avoid paying for the longterm outcome. If Medicare continues to pick up most of the cost of ESRD, prevention of kidney disease remains less likely. But if all HMO's and health insurers who "cared" for that person during the course of their diabetes were mandated to share the costs of ESRD, there would be an immediate push for early detection with microalbumin tests, and prevention with improved control and ACE inhibitors.

- Change payments for medical care from fee-for-service to fee-for-outcomes. Instead of paying for the number of visits, pay the medical staff when a person's HbA_{1c} results show their blood sugars are being controlled. If appropriate ophthalmology referrals and cholesterol tests are done, offer rewards or other incentives to the health care provider.

- Require that some part of all health care costs be paid out of pocket by the person who is being treated. The need for this financial motivation can be seen in statements like, "Oh, I don't worry how much my medicine costs, my insurance pays for everything." Real cost cutting will not occur until everyone directly feels the pinch of their own medical costs.

The greatest revelation of our generation is the discovery that human beings, by changing the inner attitudes of their minds, can change the outer aspects of their lives.

William James

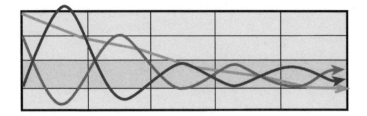

BLOOD SUGAR INVENTORY AND ACTION GUIDES

5

Recording your blood sugar readings is *the most important tool* for improving blood sugar control. Yet it is one of the hardest things for many people with diabetes to do! Recording the data needed for control takes time and commitment.

One problem is that most of the current recording methods do not provide a guide to the action choices that allow the blood sugar data that has been collected to be used to improve control. Acting upon the data collected is *the most important step* in control for most people.

In the next three chapters, we'll look at three different ways to get more usable information from your blood sugar testing.

In this chaper we'll:

- Discuss how to select targets for your blood sugars
- Introduce the Blood Sugar Inventory and Action Guides—far better than a traditional logbook
- Show how the Inventory provides a simple way to tell if your levels are normal or abnormal
- Show how to use the Action Guides to improve your blood sugar control

The Blood Sugar Inventory and Action Guides is a new product from Torrey Pines Press. You may use the ideas in this chapter as you like. To obtain the actual Inventory and Action Guides (sold as one), see order information at the back of this book.

The Inventory is a familiar logbook method to record daily blood sugar tests. But it also helps you discover when your ride on the rollercoaster is at its worst, with its patterns of highs and lows. The Action Guides are each a one-page information tool that helps you select actions to correct abnormal patterns in the readings. There are nine Action guides, each of which is designed to recommend appropriate action for a person on a specific insulin or pill regimen. You choose the one Guide that best describes your regimen. Using this two part tool over time gives you the opportunity to fine tune your results and to adapt quickly to changing circumstances.

SELECT YOUR TARGET BLOOD SUGARS

Knowing where you're going is one of the best ways of getting there. To control your blood sugars, you first want to select your target blood sugars. The target blood sugars selected will vary for different people and for different times of the day. Table 5.1 shows three typical target goals. The first column shows the target blood sugars used in the intensive control group in the Diabetes Control and Complications Trial (the group that had fewer complications). The second column shows even lower targets that are required before and during pregnancy. The third column shows higher targets that might be used by people who have Hypoglycemia Unawareness(Chapter 20).

With your physician's help, select your own premeal and postmeal target blood sugars so you can have goals to work toward. Remember, though, targets like those in the DCCT column are tight, and it takes some time for most people to achieve this degree of control even with great support!

Target Blood Sugars			
	DCCT	**Pregnant**	**Hypoglycemia Unawareness**
Before meals	70 to 120	60 to 90	100 to 180
2 hr. after meals	180 or less	120 or less*	240 or less
2-3 a.m.	over 65	60 to 90	100 to 180
HbA$_{1c}$ (if lab normal = 4-6)	less than 7.2	20% less than the upper limit for normal	less than 8

* The target blood sugar in pregnancy is 120 mg/dl at ONE hour after eating.

Table 5.1 Three Suggested Target Blood Sugars

With your physician's help, decide on your *target blood sugars*, the limits you'd like your blood sugars to stay within, for example, between 60 mg/dl and 150 mg/dl before meals (3.3 to 8.3 mmol). Fill in the blanks in Table 5.2 and then write these target blood sugars in the Inventory shown in Table 5.3.

- On the # below ___ mg/dl line, place the lowest number blood sugar should go.

- On the # above ___ mg/dl line, place the highest number blood sugar should go.

Determine Your Critical Values

Self-care has an important role in diabetes, but it is important to know when to request help. With your physician's help, decide when a blood sugar result becomes *critical*, that is, so low or so high that you should call for help. As your blood sugars (and urine ketones) rise and fall, it is important to know what single reading or pattern of readings require your physician's involvement. Knowing when to get medical help is especially important when your control is poor or when changing your routine. Recognizing "red flag" readings could even save your life!

Example: Your doctor might instruct you to call immediately if a single blood sugar reading is ever below 40 mg/dl (2.2 mmol), or if two consecutive tests are ever above 350 mg/dl (19.4 mmol) with moderate to large ketones in the urine.

Patterns Require Action

With your doctor, decide what *pattern* of high or low readings in your Inventory requires that you take acton. A pattern is a certain number of occurrences beyond your "limits" at the same time of day, say three or more readings above 160 mg/dl (8.9 mmol) before meals.

Target Blood Sugars and Critical Values

My target blood sugars are:

between _____mg/dl (mmol) and _____mg/dl(mmol) *before meals*

between _____mg/dl (mmol) and _____mg/dl (mmol) *at bedtime*

I will call my physician:

   a. for ANY reading below _____mg/dl (mmol),

   b. or more than _____ # readings above _____mg/dl (mmol)

     with ketones in the urine greater than _____ (sm, mod, lg).

Table 5.2 Fill in what you and your doctor decide are your target blood sugars and critical values.

For instance, if you had four readings before lunch during the week that were above 160 mg/dl, you would take action to correct this problem. The action might be adjusting an insulin dose, adjusting the diet or adding exerecise.

Example: To prevent frequent lows and highs, your doctor might instruct you to make an adjustment if two or more readings go below 60 mg/dl (3.3 mmol) at the same time of day, such as before dinner.

HOW TO USE THE INVENTORY (FIGURE 5.3):

1. Test your blood sugar level four times a day for a week. Fill in the Inventory completely.

2. Mark abnormal readings with an asterik (*). If you register a critically high or low reading, call your doctor as instructed.

3. Add up all the blood sugars for each period of the day that are *below* your target range. To this number, add also any insulin reactions that happened during that period of the day, whether or not a blood sugar test was done.

4. Write the total number of lows for each period of the day on lines A through D.

   Example: If in a week's time you had three low blood sugar results before dinner, plus symptoms of an insulin reaction in the afternoon (no test), place a "4" (three documented lows, plus one suspected low) on line C.

5. Add up the blood sugars before each meal and at bedtime that are *above* your target range.

6. Write the total number of high blood sugars for each day on lines E through H.

	Blood Sugar Inventory for week ____/____ to ____/____															
	Before Breakfast				**Before Lunch**			**Before Dinner**				**Before Bed**			
Date	Time	Sugar	Reg	L/N/UL	Time	Sugar	Reg	Time	Sugar	Reg	L/N/UL	Time	Sugar	Reg	L/N/UL
# below _____mg/dl	____A				____B			____C				____D			
# above _____mg/dl	____E				____F			____G				____H			
▲ Target Range	Comments:														

Record all your blood sugars for 7 days. For each time of day, count how often your readings were below and above your target range. Enter these totals in the boxes at the bottom with the letters. Then refer to these letters in your personal Action Guide for actions to reduce the number of lows & highs.

Figure 5.3 The Blood Sugar Inventory

Example: If the top of your goal is 150 mg/dl (8.3 mmol) and you had four blood sugars above this number before breakfast in the last week, write the number "4" on line E. High blood sugars "before meals" includes blood sugar readings taken 60 minutes or less before eating.

7. Circle any letter (A through H) for which the number of lows or highs is greater than your allowed limit. For instance, someone might circle the appropriate letter in the Inventory:

- When two or more low blood sugars are on lines A, B, C, or D
- Or when three or more high blood sugars on lines E, F, G, or H

Example: You may be advised by your physician to make an adjustment using your Action Guide if your blood sugar goes below 70 mg/dl (3.9 mmol) two or more times during the same period of the day over a week's time.

If you had a reading of 56 (3.1 mmol) before lunch one day and symptoms of an insulin reaction on another day at 11 a.m., you would place a "2" on line B (before lunch). Then circle B because you had two lows before lunch that week. Go to the Action Guide for advice on correcting the problem.

How To Use The Action Guide (Figure 5.9)

The Action Guides are designed for use with the Blood Sugar Inventory. Sample Action Guides are shown in Figure 5.9. Because there are many different insulin and pill regimens, a variety of Guides have been developed. There is no "one size fits all." These Action Guides cover the most common diabetes treatment plans. Use the guide that you and your physician feel best addresses your own treatment plan.

To use your Action Guide:

1. Look first for any circled letters in letters A through D in the Inventory.

2. *Stop lows first!* If letters A, B, C, or D are circled, select the letter with the largest number in it. Follow the suggestions in the Action Guide for that letter to stop the lows.

3. If letters E through H are circled (highs), select the letter with the largest number in it. Follow the suggestions in the Action Guide for that letter to stop the highs.

4. Use the Inventory to ensure the problem has been corrected. If the problem remains, try the same corrective action or try another one.

Stop Lows First

Always *stop the lows first*, particularly if your blood sugars are dropping below 50 or 60 mg/dl (2.8 to 3.3 mmol). When the blood sugar goes below 60 mg/dl, stress hormones are released. The lower the blood sugar goes and the longer it stays there, the more stress hormones are released (more

---

Tips on Using the Action Guide

Stop lows before highs.

Work first on the period of the day when the greatest number of lows or highs are happening.

If low blood sugars are either severe or frequent, do not wait a full week to lower your insulin dose! *Take action or contact your physician immediately.*

---

shaking and sweating). These stress hormones are slow to raise the blood sugar, but they may keep working to raise it for six to 10 hours after the reaction.

At any time that blood sugars go low, eat 10 to 20 grams of quick carbohydrate immediately to stop this stress hormone release and to feel better faster. Many people want to stop the reaction symptoms immediately, and may end up eating too many carbohydrates. This sends the blood sugars too high. Keep in mind that one gram of carbohydrate raises the blood sugar about four points, so 10 to 20 grams of carbohydrate are usually enough to stop a low.

If you eat more carbohydrate than 20 grams of carbohydrate, but your blood sugar does not rise, you may be taking too much insulin. However, if you are very activity, you may need to eat more than just 20 grams of carbohydrate to balance your activity.

EXAMPLES

The following examples of the Blood Sugar Inventory are typical of people with diabetes who experience too many lows, too many highs, and variable blood sugars.

Example: Low Lilly

Low Lilly checked her blood sugars for a week. Her Inventory is shown in Figure 5.4:

		Before Breakfast				Before Lunch			Before Dinner				Before Bed		
Low Lilly's Blood Sugar Inventory for week 2/6 to 2/12															
Date	Time	Sugar	Reg	L/N/UL	Time	Sugar	Reg	Time	Sugar	Reg	L/N/UL	Time	Sugar	Reg	L/N/UL
2/6	7:15	99	4	23	12:00	153		6:00	77	7	3	10:50	46 ✳		
2/7	8:30	83	4	23	12:30	138		5:30	111	7	3	10:30	83		
2/8	8:30	143	5	23	12:45	105		5:30	84	7	3	10:45	31 ✳		
2/9	8:30	136	4	23	12:30	152		6:20	69	7	3	11:30	104		
2/10	8:15	83	4	23	12:45	58		5:30	137	7	3	10:50	56 ✳		
2/11	8:20	112	4	23	12:15	102		5:45	103	7	3	10:45	64		
2/12	7:30	96	4	23	11:45	124		6:00	201	9	3	9:50	73		
# below 60 mg/dl	__A				_1__B			__C				③_D			
# above 170 mg/dl	__E				__F			_1__G				__H			
Target Range	Comments:														

Figure 5.4 Low Lilly's Blood Sugar Inventory

After filling out her Inventory, Lilly noticed the frequent lows at bedtime (marked with an asterik *) and circled their total at letter D on her Inventory. After checking her Action Guide, she realized she was getting too much Regular for dinner. She lowered her dinner Regular from 7 units to 6 units to stop these lows.

Whenever frequent or severe low blood sugars occur, insulin doses must be cut.

Think of two reasons why your blood sugar might be going low. Write these reasons down along with what you can do to reduce these lows:

Reason #1: _____

What I can do: _____

Reason #2: _____

What I can do: _____

Example: **High Hank** checked his sugars for a week. His results are found in Figure 5.5.

High Hank's Blood Sugar Inventory for week 9/11 to 9/17															
	Before Breakfast				Before Lunch			Before Dinner				Before Bed			
Date	Time	Sugar	Reg	L/N/UL	Time	Sugar	Reg	Time	Sugar	Reg	L/N/UL	Time	Sugar	Reg	L/N/UL
9/11	7:15	99	6	32	12:00	153	2	6:00	77	7	10	10:50	96		
9/12	8:30	83	6	32	12:30	178✳	3	5:30	111	7	10	10:30	133		
9/13	8:30	143	7	32	12:30	197✳	4	5:30	84	7	10	10:45	95		
9/14	8:30	136	7	32	12:45	152✳	2	6:20	69	7	10	11:30	104		
9/15	8:15	83	6	32	12:15	218✳	4	5:30	137	7	10	10:50	153		
9/16	8:20	112	6	32	12:30	185	2	5:45	103	7	10	10:45	87		
9/17	7:30	96	6	32	11:45	147		6:00	171	9	10	9:50	75		
# below 70 mg/dl	___A				___B			_1_C				___D			
# above 160 mg/dl	___E				④_F			_1_G				___H			
Target Range	Comments: Felt "dopey" after breakfast all week!														

Figure 5.5 High Hank's Blood Sugar Inventory

After seeing this pattern of high readings at lunch (F), Hank circled F because four occurrences were outside his acceptable range. Then he checked his Action Guide. He decided that he would eat less carbohydrate for breakfast because he also wanted to lose some weight.

Tips On Insulin Adjustments

1. Under most circumstances, change only one insulin at a time

2. Allow at least three to four days before making another adjustment, unless your blood sugars are very very high or very low.

3. Change doses by one or two units, or up to 10 percent of your total daily insulin dose. For example, somone having frequent lows on a daily total of 50 units of insulin might need to reduce their doses by up to five units (10% of 50 units).

4. Be conservative. Make one change at a time. Wait to see what effect this has before making another change.

Example: Complex Carl was having a lot of ups and downs. His Inventory (Figure 5.6) showed the following data:

Complex Carl's Blood Sugar Inventory for week 7/16 to 7/22															
	Before Breakfast				Before Lunch			Before Dinner				Before Bed			
Date	Time	Sugar	Reg	L/N/UL	Time	Sugar	Reg	Time	Sugar	Reg	L/N/UL	Time	Sugar	Reg	L/N/UL
7/16	7:15	72	4	38	12:00	121		6:00	57	6	10	9:50	287		
7/17	6:30	✳ 87	4	38	11:30	153		5:30	109	7	10	9:30	141		
7/18	5:30	61 ✳	4	38	"	97		5:30	90	7	10	9:45	87		
7/19	6:30	90	4	38	"	106		6:20	47	6	10	10:30	211		
7/20	4:30	53 ✳	3	38	"	207	2	5:30	131	7	10	9:50	164		
7/21	6:20	46 ✳	3	38	:	191	1	5:45	110	7	10	9:45	78		
7/22	7:30	78	4	38	12:45	124		6:00	*73	9	10	10:50	77		
# below 70 mg/dl	④_A				___B			_3_C				___D			
# above 160 mg/dl	___E				_3_F			___G				_3_H			
Target Range	Comments: *Woke up in a sweat at 3AM on the 17th and ate. Low in the afternoon on the 22nd.														

Figure 5.6 Complex Carl's Blood Sugar Inventory

At 3 A.M. on the morning of the 17th, Carl had an insulin reaction. Though he didn't test his blood sugar, Carl counted the reaction on his Inventory that morning before breakfast. With the 3 lows that happened before breakfast on other days and the low during the night, Carl had four lows before breakfast (A). Before dinner, he had two lows, and with an afternoon reaction on another day, he had a total of three lows before dinner (C).

Carl also had three highs before lunch (F) and three more before bed (H). He noted that his low blood sugars were usually before breakfast and dinner. His highs were before lunch and at bedtime. Carl decided take take these three actions after consulting his Action Guide:

1. He treated the lows first. For the lows before breakfast (A), Carl lowered his dinner Lente from 10 to 8 units. He decided to also eat a small bedtime snack to lessen the chances for lows during the night. Because of the nighttime low, he set his alarm for 2 A.M. for two nights to make sure he wasn't having nighttime reactions and sleeping through them.

2. For the lows before dinner (C), he decreased his breakfast Lente from 38 to 36 units to lessen the amount of insulin working in the afternoon.

3. For the highs before lunch and bed (F&H), Carl didn't do anything. He noticed that most of these highs followed lows and that he might simply be eating too much to treat his lows. He decided to try stopping his lows first and to be careful not to overeat if he was low.

Example: No Pattern Patty shows no clear pattern in her Blood Sugar Inventory (Fig. 5.7):

No Pattern Patty's Blood Sugar Inventory for week 5/2 to 5/8																
	Before Breakfast				Before Lunch			Before Dinner				Before Bed			
Date	Time	Sugar	Reg	L/N/UL	Time	Sugar	Reg	Time	Sugar	Reg	L/N/UL	Time	Sugar	Reg	L/N/UL
5/2	9:15	72	5	26	12:00	183	3	5:15	50	7	3	9:50	259		
5/3	6:30	47	4	20	11:30	153		5:30	241	9	3	9:30	233		
5/4	6:20	287	10	26	2:30	38		5:30	319	11	3	11:45	34		
5/5	8:30	192	7	26	12:45	211		5:20	41	0	0	9:30	324		
5/6	6:15	62	0	26	1:00	308	2	5:30	122	7	3	9:50	186		
5/7	6:20	153	6	26	11:00	55		5:15	203	7	3	1:00	137		
5/8	9:30	80	4	26	12:45	124		7:00	79	7	3	9:50	73		
# below 60 mg/dl	(1) A				(2) B			(2) C				(1) D			
# above 170 mg/dl	(2) E				(3) F			(3) G				(4) H			
Target Range	Comments: Felt tired all week. Really bad ups and downs for no reason!														

Figure 5.7 No Pattern Patty's Blood Sugar Inventory

Here, lows and highs are happening at all times of the day. Patty couldn't use the Action Guide because there was no clear pattern to her blood sugars.

Patty realized three things. She was eating at different times of the day because of demands at work. Sometimes she skipped her insulin or meals altogether. And she really wasn't on a meal plan.

She phoned her physician, who made a referral to the dietician for help on balancing her meals and counting carbohydrates. The dietician also helped Patty decide on how much insulin to take for the various situations she was encountering, and to set up a High Blood Sugar Regular or Sliding Scale for situations in which her blood sugar was high.

After taking these actions to stop her ups and downs, Patty planned to do her Inventory again in another week, and then consider whether further action was needed.

Why Does The Blood Sugar Go:	
Too High?	**Too Low?**
a large meal	a light meal
snacking	a missed meal
less exercise	eating late
extra stress	more exercise
too little insulin	too much insulin

Figure 5.8 Reasons Why The Blood Sugar Goes Too High And Too Low

		Blood Sugar Action Guide #2		
		For those on Regular before breakfast, lunch, and dinner, plus a long-acting insulin in AM and PM		
Letter	Problem	Insulin Choice	Food Choice	Exercise Choice
A	Lows at night or before breakfast	Lower evening L/N/UL. If night lows happen within 7 hrs. of taking dinner Regular, consider lowering it.	Eat a bedtime snack with more carbs and some protein	Less exercise is usually not recommended as a choice, unless your activity is quite strenuous.
B	Lows between breakfast and lunch	Lower breakfast Regular. If low at A&B, lower evening L/N/UL.	Eat more carbs at breakfast or add a midmorning snack	
C	Lows between lunch and dinner	Lower lunch Regular or morning L/N/UL.	Eat more carbs at lunch or add an afternoon snack	
D	Lows between dinner and bedtime	Lower dinner Regular.	Eat more carbs at dinner or add an after dinner snack	
E	Highs before breakfast	Raise evening L/N/UL. Move L/N to bedtime? Change UL to L or N?	Eat less at dinner or for a bedtime snack	Increase evening exercise
F	Highs before lunch	Raise morning Regular.	Eat less at breakfast or for midmorning snack	Increase morning exercise
G	Highs before dinner	Raise lunch Regular or morning L/N/UL.	Eat less at lunch or for afternoon snack	Increase afternoon exercise
H	Highs before bed	Raise dinner Regular.	Eat less at dinner, or snack less during the evening	Increase evening exercise

Discuss with your physician any changes in medication or insulin BEFORE taking action

		Blood Sugar Action Guide #7A		
		For those on Regular and a long-acting insulin before dinner, plus a diabetes pill before breakfast		
Letter	Problem	Insulin Choice	Food Choice	Exercise Choice
A	Lows at night or before breakfast	Lower dinner L/N/UL. If nighttime lows happen within 7 hrs. of taking dinner Regular, consider lowering it.	Eat a bedtime snack with more carbs and some protein	Less exercise is usually not recommended as a choice, unless your activity is quite strenuous.
B	Lows between breakfast and lunch	Lower dinner L/N/UL or reduce dose of morning diabetes pill.	Eat more carbs at breakfast or add a midmorning snack	
C	Lows between lunch and dinner	Reduce dose of morning diabetes pill.	Eat more carbs at lunch or add an afternoon snack	
D	Lows between dinner and bedtime	Lower dinner Regular.	Eat more carbs at dinner or add an after dinner snack	
E	Highs before breakfast	Raise dinner L/N/UL. Move L/N to bedtime? If on UL, change to L or N.	Eat less at dinner or in the bedtime snack	Increase evening exercise
F	Highs before lunch	Raise dose of morning diabetes pill, or start morning insulin.	Eat less at breakfast or in the midmorning snack	Increase morning exercise
G	Highs before dinner	Raise dose of morning diabetes pill, or start morning insulin.	Eat less at lunch or in the afternoon snack	Increase afternoon exercise
H	Highs before bed	Raise dinner Regular.	Eat less at dinner, or snack less during the evening	Increase evening exercise

Discuss with your physician any changes in medication or insulin BEFORE taking action

Figure 5.9 Two of the Action Guides

If your project doesn't work,
look for the part that you didn't think was important.
Arthur Block

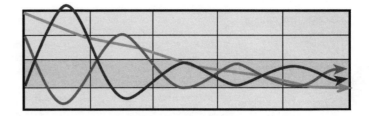

SMART CHARTS—BETTER CONTROL AT A GLANCE

6

A normal blood sugar is the result of insulin entering the bloodstream in the correct amount and at the right time to balance other factors that raise or lower it (carbohydrates, activity, stress, etc.). Charting all these factors does take some time and effort, *but it is the best way to get a complete picture of all the information needed for control.*

In this chapter, we'll show how to use a superior charting system, called Smart Charts. In the next chapter, Timothy Bailey, M.D., will describe how to use some of the latest meter and computer technology to bring meaning to your numbers. Then in the chapters that follow, we'll show you how to use this information to stop the rollercoaster and gain better control.

This chapter describes:

- Why charting is important
- How to make a chart
- An example of a completed chart

WHY BOTHER USING A CHART?

Your lifestyle changes. Days lengthen and shorten, activity increases and decreases, weekends differ from weekdays, food intake shifts from more carbohydrate in the summer to more fat in the winter. All of these affect insulin need and blood sugar levels. Good charts allow you to identify when and where insulin adjustments are needed.

Compared to traditional logbooks, charts reveal at a glance whether your blood sugars are above or below your desired range. They reveal the time of day problems occur. They let you collect in one place everything affecting your control. They reveal all of this in a graphical format which shows the rise and fall of your blood sugars.

Over time, charts tell you if you are getting where you want to go. They become your guide, letting you know whether the changes you make are really helping you gain better control. Charts allow you to visualize the patterns in your readings, such as any consistent rise or fall of the blood sugars. These patterns may show that you have frequent lows in the afternoon, that your readings are running high most of the time, that eating certain meals or eating at a particular restaurant causes your blood sugars to go high or low, or that stress or a change in weight has affected your readings. As you gather this information on your charts, patterns become apparent. Some typical blood sugar patterns and what to do about them are discussed in Chapters 24 through 28.

The discipline required in charting leads to freedom from the worry of unknown internal damage, freedom from the annoyance and frustration of blood sugar test results that are always out of control, and freedom from the rollercoaster mood swings caused by high and low blood sugars. Most importantly, the person who charts gains the freedom to eat, work and exercise the way he or she wants.

A charting format called a "Smart Chart" is used in this book and a blank Smart Chart is shown below. You may order a supply of Smart Charts from the back page of this book. Smart Charts are a perfect size to slip into a checkbook cover for easy carrying in your pocket or purse.

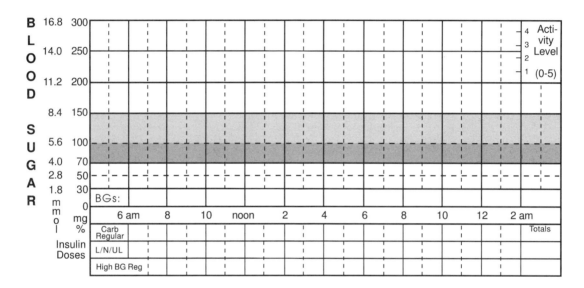

Figure 6.1 The Smart Chart provides optimal information in a handy checkbook size format.

WHAT DO I PUT ON MY SMART CHART?

The more information you place on your charts, the easier it becomes to control your blood sugars. Particularly important are blood sugar readings, carbohydrate intake, insulin doses, periods of exercise and periods of stress. Keep Smart Charts or a data collection device handy for quick access. Most people find charting easier if they carry their charts with them.

To identify patterns and problem areas, record the following items on your Smart Charts:

Activity Levels

Record your physical activity, exercise or work in the *activity level area* at the top of the graph. See Figure 6.2. Put down any activity that's greater than your usual daily activity. For instance, if you golf only on Saturdays, you would want to record it. Occasional activities like this often have to be balanced with extra carbohydrate or a reduction in insulin doses. On the other hand, if you run 5 miles at the same time every day, this is normal daily activity for you and probably requires no change in your usual daily routine once a correct insulin adjustment has been established.

Rank your physical activity on a 1 to 5 scale. A "1" indicates a *mild increase* in activity, while a "5" would be given to activities that are *strenuous*. For instance, if sitting behind a desk is your usual work activity, but you spend the day moving your files and records to a new office, you would record a "1," "3," or "5" during the appropriate workday hours, based on how much work this moving required.

If you begin a running program and become quite winded during this new exercise, you would graph a "5" on your chart at the time of the run. After you run for a few days or weeks, this same run may no longer be strenuous for you and then would be listed as a "4" or a "3."

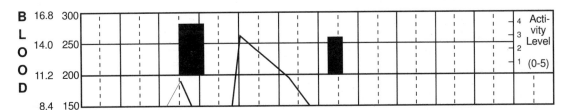

Figure 6.2 Activity Levels: Bicycling for an hour and 15 minutes (level 4) in the morning, loading dirt into a trailer (level 3) for 45 minutes that afternoon.

Blood Sugar Readings

Graphing blood sugar readings reveals blood sugar patterns. Recognizing these patterns helps you manage your sugar levels more effectively. The minimum number of tests needed to adjust insulin doses is four a day: before each meal and at bedtime. Additional information is gained by testing two hours after meals. A complete picture of blood sugar patterns can be obtained with seven tests a day. Occasionally, a test at 2 a.m. is also needed. The boxes in the middle of the chart just below the blood sugar graphing area are for recording *blood sugar readings* and *insulin reactions*. See Figure 6.3

Test your blood sugar whenever low blood sugar symptoms occur, unless the symptoms are severe enough that waiting to test would be dangerous. If severe symptoms occur, test as quickly as possible after eating or ask someone else to test you. It's important to check your blood sugar if you feel low. Other conditions, such as excitement, fatigue, stress or anxiety can mimic the symptoms of a low blood sugar. An exact blood sugar measurement allows you to take precise corrective action.

The *time* of all insulin reactions should be marked on the charts regardless of whether a blood sugar test was done. Indicate all verified or suspected insulin reactions on the chart with

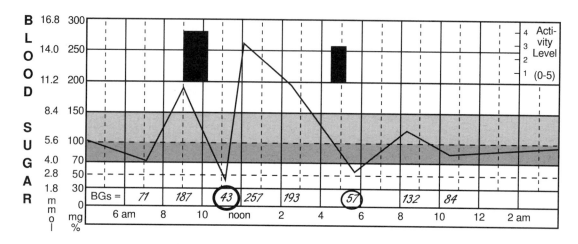

Figure 6.3 Blood sugar readings. Low blood sugars with symptoms (circled readings) are shown at 11 a.m. and 5:30 p.m.

a circle. It also helps to record the severity of these reactions. For instance, if symptoms are mild, use a small circle. With severe symptoms, use a large circle.

The first step to better blood sugar control is eliminating severe or frequent insulin reactions. Identifying the pattern in which they occur makes prevention possible.

Insulin Doses

On the lines in the middle of your chart, record your long-acting and Regular insulin doses, and the time at which they were taken. Lines are provided for each of the three insulin doses: the long-acting insulin, Carb Regular, and High Blood Sugar Regular. See Figure 6.4.

		6 am	8	10	noon	2	4	6	8	10	12	2 am	
Insulin Doses	Carb Regular	6		2	6		8						Totals 20
	L/N/UL	10								8			18
	High BG Reg				2								4
													42

Figure 6.4 Insulin Doses. Chart shows doses given at 8 a.m., noon, 5 p.m., and 10 p.m. with the day's totals on the right.

Food List And Carbohydrate Content

Carbohydrate is the principle ingredient in foods that raises the blood sugar. Counting carbs directly from a label or indirectly by measuring food exchanges is relatively easy to do. It also makes sense. For the first time, you are measuring *the part of food that influences your blood sugars.* See Chapter 8 to learn how to count carbs.

Measure and record all the carbohydrates you eat. Consult with your dietician to obtain a precise recommendation for your own carbohydrate need, as well as information on ways to improve your blood sugars and health through your food choices.

Once the total daily carbohydrate intake is determined, it is divided into the number of grams you plan to eat for each meal and snack during the day. The amount of carbohydrate you want at each meal and snack can be tailored to fit your own schedule and food preferences. Your personal ratio of Regular to carbohydrate can be determined to allow varied meal sizes.

At the bottom of the chart, identify each food eaten, the time, and the amount of carbohydrate it contains. Figure 6.5 shows an example. *Be specific.* A general word like "cereal" won't do as all cereals are not equal. Cheerios®, Grape Nuts®, corn flakes, and oatmeal have very different effects on the blood sugars. Writing "sandwich" down is very different from "sandwich: whole wheat/tuna/mayo, 32 grams." This is also very different from "sandwich: ice cream, 68 grams."

Only by listing exactly what you eat and the exact amount of carbohydrate the food contains can you determine the effect these foods are having on your blood sugars. You will likely find that some foods have undesired effects on your blood sugars, while others thought to be "bad" may be perfectly fine.

Don't overlook what you eat to correct low blood sugars. If you don't record the four graham crackers (44 grams) and 16 ounces of milk (24 grams) that you took for a nighttime reaction, you won't remember why your blood sugar was 307 mg/dl (17.1 mmol) the next morning.

List all foods, not just carbohydrates. You may discover that foods with little carbohydrate, like cheese or nuts, cause your blood sugar to climb gradually for several hours after you eat them. It helps if you also estimate how much of these foods you've eaten. List amounts, like two ounces of cheese or 10 ounces of prime rib, on your charts.

Breakfast			**Lunch**			**Dinner**		
Time	Food	Carb grams	Time	Food	Carb grams	Time	Food	Carb grams
7:30	1 cup milk NF	13	1:00	1 cup milk NF	13	6:00	pasta and clams	70
	Cheerios 64 gr	46		tuna sandwich	36		green salad	8
	2 rye toast	30		apple 154 grams	23		Chardonnay	6
	strawberries	12		ginger snap cookie	6		vanilla ice cream	20
	poached egg	0						
		101			78			104
Morning Snacks			Afternoon Snacks			Evening Snacks		
11:00	2 blueberry muffins	70	5:30	glucose tabs	10	10:30	peaches	16
	banana	25		cheese and crackers	16		cottage cheese	14
		95			26			30

Figure 6.5 Food list with carbohydrate content in grams

Emotions, Stress, And Other Comments

In the comments section at the top of your Smart Chart, record any other information you feel is relevant. See Figure 6.6. Emotions, stress and illness can all affect blood sugars. This information might be "I have a cold," or "I woke up with a headache and may have had a reaction during the night." The high blood sugar before dinner could be explained by a comment that "work was very stressful that day."

Emotions and blood sugars are a two-way street. Understanding these connections can help in your blood sugar control. The brain controls the secretion of various stress hormones which interfere with insulin. The brain, however, depends entirely on blood sugar for fuel. When either high or low levels of sugar reach the brain, the response can be loss of memory, anger, irritability, slowed thinking or depression.

As blood sugars rise, hormones that prevent depression are lowered. When depressed, a person has less energy to do the things needed for good control: thoughtful selection of foods, regular exercise and rest. As you can see, it becomes a vicious cycle that needs to be broken. The Comments section is the place to begin connecting your own emotions and blood sugars.

Day: *Saturday*	Comments:	*Great AM ride--rode 17 miles! Starved and ate LOTS!*
Date: *4 / 27 / 96*		*noon: VERY grouchy at nursery 4:30 PM--helped Bob load dirt*
© 1994, Diabetes Services, Inc.		

Figure 6.6 Comments help you see how events affect your readings

BLOOD SUGAR PATTERNS

As you look over completed Smart Charts, you will notice a pattern of high and low blood sugars. Set aside a time each week to look for patterns. For instance, every Saturday morning review the last seven days' charts.

Look for patterns that show the time of day when the following situations occur

- High blood sugars or insulin reactions
- Drops in blood sugars due to exercise
- High or low blood sugars following particular foods
- High blood sugars following insulin reactions
- Differences between weekend and workday blood sugars

Show your charts to others. Listen to suggestions from family and friends. Diabetes personnel in particular understand the complexities of diabetes in daily life. Seek the knowledge and experience of others to shorten and simplify your path toward normal readings. Another person, especially someone trained in diabetes care, will see things that you miss. If you have any uncertainty about a potential pattern or the need to adjust your insulin, be sure to contact your physician/health care team for advice. Use these specialists to make your work easier.

Data collected in your Smart Charts may be more extensive than you normally need. But charting the factors that influence your blood sugars allows you to understand and change them. After you stabilize your blood sugar, a simple daily log may be all you need. If, in the future, you suspect you are back on the rollercoaster, going back to the Smart Charts should help you regain control.

A SAMPLE CHART

On the next page is a completed Smart Chart for Chris who is on flexible insulin therapy. See Figure 6.7. Read the background information about Chris, then take a look at his one day chart. Decide for yourself what you would do if you were Chris and this were your chart. What's happening to his blood sugars? Why? What would you do about it? Write your suggestions down on paper. After giving Chris' chart some thought about the changes you would make, look over the analysis that follows for confirmation of your thinking. Don't peek!

Chris' Background:

Chris is 32 years old and has had diabetes for 18 years. He has been on flexible insulin therapy for three years. He weighs 156 pounds and leads an active lifestyle, eating about 2200 calories a day with half of these calories coming from carbohydrate. He tests his blood sugar four to six times a day and counts carbohydrates for diet control. During the day, he usually eats 75 grams of carbohydrate for breakfast, 90 grams for lunch and an afternoon snack, and 110 grams for dinner.

His control has been good. Chris and his physician have agreed on target blood sugars between 70 and 130 mg/dl (3.9 to 7.2 mmol) before meals and under 160 mg/dl (9.3 mmol) after meals. He uses one unit of Regular for every 13 grams of carbohydrate that he eats. For high blood sugars, he takes one unit of Regular for every 40 points above 100 mg/dl before meals. He normally uses glucose tablets to treat his insulin reactions.

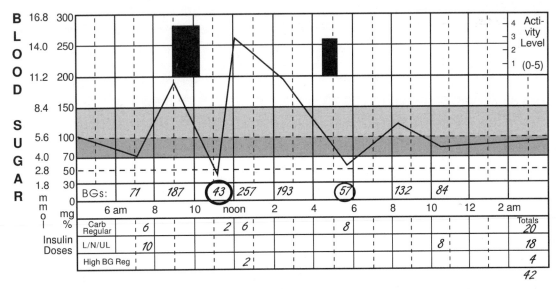

Breakfast			Lunch			Dinner		
Time	Food	Carb grams	Time	Food	Carb grams	Time	Food	Carb grams
7:30	1 cup milk NF	13	1:00	1 cup milk NF	13	6:00	pasta and clams	70
	Cheerios 64 gr	46		tuna sandwich	36		green salad	8
	2 rye toast	30		apple 154 grams	23		Chardonnay	6
	strawberries	12		ginger snap cookie	6		vanilla ice cream	20
	poached egg	0						
		101			78			104

Morning Snacks			Afternoon Snacks			Evening Snacks		
11:00	2 blueberry muffins	70	5:30	glucose tabs	10	10:30	peaches	16
	banana	25		cheese and crackers	16		cottage cheese	14
		95			26			30

Day: *Saturday*
Date: *4 | 27 | 96*
© 1994, Diabetes Services, Inc.

Comments: *Great AM ride--rode 17 miles! Starved and ate LOTS!*
noon: VERY grouchy at nursery 4:30 PM--helped Bob load dirt

Figure 6.7 One Day's Smart Chart for Chris

ANALYSIS:

In looking at Chris' chart, you can see his blood sugars bounced quite a bit on this day. Because it's a weekend he is more active and he tested his blood sugar frequently. His readings averaged in the normal range, with the first and last sugars absolutely normal, but five of eight blood sugar tests were out of his desired range.

He takes his evening dose of eight units of Lente at bedtime because of nighttime reactions in the past. Because his blood sugar dropped from 128 mg/dl (7.1 mmol) at 3 a.m. that morning (not shown) to 71 mg/dl (3.9 mmol) at 7 a.m. before breakfast, his bedtime dose may still be slightly too high.

Chris' food choices are balanced with a variety of foods. He took six units of Regular 30 minutes before breakfast. Since he uses one unit for each 13 grams, this would normally cover 78 grams of carbohydrate. He ate 101 grams for breakfast, intending the extra 23 grams to help offset his bike ride later that morning. The blood sugar at 9 a.m. of 187 mg/dl (10.4 mmol) at an hour and a half after breakfast reflects this reduced coverage.

Chris took an extended bike ride of 17½ miles in an hour and 15 minutes (averaging 14 miles per hour). This exercise will use at most 83 grams of carbohydrate each hour, or 104 grams for the whole bike ride. His extra 23 grams eaten at breakfast was not enough carbohydrate to cover this ride.

The low blood sugar at 11 a.m. following the ride was caused by this lack of carbs. Unfortunately, when the insulin reaction occurred, Chris overate, having two medium-sized blueberry muffins (35 grams each) and a banana (25 grams). The food, plus the stress hormones released by the insulin reaction (a large circle indicates a major reaction), caused his blood sugar to rise sharply to 257 mg/dl (14.3 mmol).

As his appetite subsided and he realized he had overeaten, he partly corrected the excess carbohydrate with an extra injection of two units of Regular, enough to cover 26 grams of these excess carbohydrates.

In his comments, Chris notes that he felt "very grouchy" at noon. This irritability happened as his blood sugar was spiking to the mid-200 range and might be due to his high blood sugar.

At lunch, he took extra High Blood Sugar Regular to lower the reading. He wanted to be at 100 mg/dl (5.6 mmol), so he subtracted 100 from 257 to get his desired drop of 157 (or 8.7 mmol). Since he drops 40 points (2.2 mmol) per unit, he would normally take four extra units to bring the blood sugar down. Instead, he took only two extra units of Regular for the high reading because most of the previous two units he had taken at 11:15 a.m. still had to work. On these two units, plus the six units of Regular for lunch, his blood sugar dropped to 193 two hours after lunch.

His neighbor, Bob, got him to volunteer to shovel dirt into a trailer that afternoon. Because this activity wasn't planned, he didn't eat extra food before starting to shovel. A mild low blood sugar followed at 5:30 and he covered it with 10 grams of glucose tablets, plus cheese and crackers. Dinner was covered well by 8 units of Regular, with great readings of 132 mg/dl (7.3 mmol) 2 hours after dinner and 84 mg/dl (4.7 mmol) at bedtime.

WHAT CHRIS LEARNED FROM HIS SMART CHARTS

When he analyzed his charts with his health provider, Chris agreed to:

- Use less evening Lente to ease the nighttime drop in his blood sugar, then retest the new dose to see if it keeps the overnight blood sugar stable.

- Estimate more accurately the extra carbohydrate needed to cover activities like cycling and shovelling dirt. Before his bike ride or a half hour into the ride, he could have had a banana along with a cup of milk (approximately 37 grams total), along with another 40 grams or so of carbohydrate fluids during the ride. From the chart, this 77 grams along with the extra 17 grams taken at breakfast probably would have covered the ride. (104 grams equals the maximum need)

- Make note of any relationship between irritability and blood sugars. If this is a pattern, recognizing it may avoid some embarrassing personal encounters in the future.

- Always use fast carbohydrate for reactions. Products like glucose tablets and honey raise the blood sugar quickly and decrease the amount of stress hormones released into the blood. When the blood sugar rises to normal faster, more rational decisions can be made that prevent overeating.

- Be sure to add a bedtime snack when activity levels are higher than usual that day. Extra physical activity can lower the blood sugar for 24 hours or more.

SOME FINAL TIPS

As you first start filling out the Smart Charts, you may find it difficult to record all of this information. However, by carrying charts with you and making sure to record insulin doses and foods regularly, you'll find it much easier to correct any problems you may run into as you begin to improve your control. With practice, charting becomes a small daily effort that can yield big payoffs.

Get in the habit of reviewing your charts regularly for patterns, as well as sharing this information with your physician/health care team. We analyzed only one day's Smart Chart here due to space restrictions, but you will usually review at least a week's worth of charts to find your own patterns.

If your charts are loose, make it a habit to lay them side by side or top to bottom at least once a week. If bound together, analyze them by flipping back and forth. Looking over your charts regularly will help you recognize and improve your blood sugar patterns, keep blood sugars as normal as possible, and maximize your good health.

Take notes on the spot, a note is worth a cart-load of recollections.

Ralph Waldo Emerson

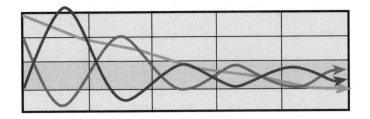

CHARTING WITH COMPUTERS
AN EASY GUIDE TO DATA MANAGEMENT

BY TIMOTHY S. BAILEY, M.D., F.A.C.P., F.A.C.E.

7

Are you taking full advantage of all the high-tech features that your blood sugar meter has to offer? Have you considered using your computer to help you track your blood sugars? With today's high tech meters and a basic computer, you can easily record the data you need for control and then download it to your computer for analysis in a matter of minutes. Once downloaded, this information can be printed in graphs and charts that help you pinpoint changes that will improve your blood sugars. You save time and effort, and you know the data is going to help you.

This chapter will discuss:

- How to collect data from a glucose meter
- How to organize the data
- How to find trends and patterns
- How to use graphs and charts to provide an accurate record

You may already be keeping a conventional logbook. In the previous chapters, we presented a superior way to keep logs and charting trends in The Blood Sugar Inventory and Action Guides and in Smart Charts. If one of these methods works well for you, you don't need a computer.

However, you may find that a computer is able to analyze and present data in superior ways. This can be a real win-win situation for you and your health providers. You may appreciate their timesaving ability. Your health care providers will also appreciate your presentation of data in an accesible way. If this is the case, computer charting is quite likely the method for you.

COLLECTING DATA: THE HARDWARE

Computers that will work best with today's glucose programs are IBM compatible with at least a 386sx processor, running Microsoft Windows 3.1, Windows 95, or OS/2 Warp. Also required are a 1.44 MB 3½ inch floppy disk drive, a mouse or trackball, and a VGA or better monitor.

Glucose meters can work with your computer to provide detailed analysis of your blood sugar data. To do this, you must have a meter that has memory to record both the blood sugar readings and the time the test was made. More advanced meters can also remember and analyse data such as insulin doses, carbohydrate counts, activity levels and special "events" such as insulin reactions or extra stress.

Meters currently available in early 1996 and their capabilities are listed in Table 7.1. These meters differ in the technology used to measure the blood sugar and in how extra data is entered in those meters that have this capability. You will want to try out any meter before purchase because each differs in ease of use and ease of collecting additional data.

Brand/Model	Memory	Events	Insulin	Diet	Exercise	Call
Accu-Chek® Advantage	100					(800) 858-8072
Accu-Check® Easy	350	✓				(800) 858-8072
Bayer® Glucometer-M	300	✓	✓	✓	✓	(800) 348-8100
Cascade® Checkmate Plus	255		✓			(800) 525-6718
Medisense® Precision	125					(800) 527-3339
One Touch Profile™	250	✓	✓	✓	✓	(800) 227-8862

Table 7.1 Current meters and their features

Connector Cables which link the meter and computer are sold by most meter manufacturers for between $5 (LifeScan® meter) and $140 (MediSense® meter). You need a cable specially built for each brand of meter. This cable connects to a plug in the back of your computer called the "serial port." This port is a RS232 com port often found near the printer port and is required for the transfer of data. Depending upon your computer, you may also need a 9 to 25 pin converter. The converter costs about $5 and changes the size of the serial port to adapt to the cable from the meter company.

Macintosh owners will need the same kind of cable used for an "external modem."

COLLECTING DATA: THE SOFTWARE

Once you are ready to connect you need a software program to the meter and turn it into intelligible ments. Insist on a 30-day money-gram you try, as the quality of the able.

your meter to your computer, download the raw data from graphs, charts and other docu-back guarantee for any pro-products offered is quite vari-

Although IBM users currently options, MAC afficionadoes will only macros, or hypercard stacks available

have a number of software find spreadsheet templates, for downloading data.

Glucose meter corporations (such as Boehringer Mannheim®, Bayer®, LifeScan®, MediSense® and Cascade Medical®) have produced software programs which are sold exclusively for their meters. These programs have often been designed for use by physicians, and are not currently being used by any significant number of doctors or patients. They are impractical in settings where different brands of meters are being used, such as a physician's office or in a home in which different brands of meters are being used.

The Internet offers many patient-developed applications ranging from simple spreadsheet templates to shareware with more features. These are inexpensive or free, but provide only rudimentary graphing and charting. You can find some of these programs in the "Meters & Testing" library in the "Diabetes Forum" on the Compuserve online information service. Also, you can check out diabetes-related "web sites" with a browser. See the on-line resources listed at the end of this chapter.

Commercial software generally offers a more polished product. One of the leaders in software to download meters is MetaMedix.™ Their Mellitus Manager® software offers the most comprehensive approach to charting information from meters. E-mail may be sent to MetaMedix at 70410.754@compuserve.com, or viewed with a browser at http://www.diabetesnet.com.

On all software, check out the technical support available and be sure there is a return policy on purchases. As yet, no software program has become an industry standard. Your diabetes educator can be a helpful resource for separating the wheat from the chaff.

HOW SOFTWARE ORGANIZES THE DATA

The two basic ways to organize data are the logbook and the chart. The logbook is merely a detailed record of your readings, the time tested, your food intake and insulin reactions. To create a chart without a computer, you usually have to create a logbook first. With a computer, both logbooks and charting become easier.

Depending on the software you have chosen, the data collected from your glucose meter may appear as columns of numbers. You can print these columns to make up a logbook. The advantage here is that the computer prints the data entered directly from the meter. You don't have to write it all out by hand as with a conventional logbook.

A chart gives you an added advantage in being able to see at a glance how your blood sugars are doing. You can quickly see if you are meeting your goals or if you are skating on thin ice. Most software programs allow you to view the same material as a bar graph, a pie graph or a line graph. If you are creative, you can devise your own style of graph and print it out in glorious color. You can also use your own humorous clip art to comment on your progress.

CREATING YOUR COMPUTER CHART

Let's say you have a glucose meter that stores information about blood sugar tests, insulin doses, and carbohydrates eaten (in grams). Into your software program you put the goals of diabetes care and improvement that you and your health care team have decided on. Attach your meter to the computer and you're ready to go!

Logbook Options

A statistics report provides information about your averages; your readings above and below your target goals; low blood sugar occurances and events. The statistics report can show the number of times during the day that blood sugars fall below your hypoglycemic threshold. You can find average values of readings related to certain events, such as exercise.

A report is the familiar logbook format with columns running horizontally and vertically. Each reading and insulin dose is recorded by mealtimes. The report is a simple way to display information. Although you must study the report a bit, you can discover trends and patterns. Some software programs offer enhanced logbook options, such as the one on the next page with a thumbnail graphic that shows each day's blood sugar pattern.

Tue 8/22/95		7:15 a	10:25 a	12:13 p	3:58 p	5:58 p	8:03 p	11:53 p		
Glucose		268	176	115	37	239	182	123		
N / R	-/-	25/18+2	-/-	-/0	-/-	20/15	-/-	-/0	-/-	-/-
grams CHO / Exercise (min)	-/-	56/-	-/-	82/-	65/65	60/-	-/-	52/-	-/-	-/-
Event1 / Event2	-/-	-/-	-/-	-/-	-/-	-/-	-/-	-/-	-/-	-/-
Comments										
Wed 8/23/95		7:23 a	8:44 a	11:44 a	2:02 p	6:27 p	8:41 p	10:56 p		
Glucose		334	219	53	41	119	176	136		
N / R	-/-	25/18+2	-/-	-/0	-/-	20/15	-/-	-/0	-/-	-/-
grams CHO / Exercise (min)	-/-	-/-	60/-	50/-	45/-	90/55	32/-	12/-	-/-	-/-
Event1 / Event2	-/-	-/-	-/-	-/-	-/-	-/-	-/-	-/-	-/-	-/-
Comments										
Thu 8/24/95		8:08 a	10:57 a	12:33 p	3:06 p	6:33 p	8:48 p	10:59 p		
Glucose		205	117	134	51	119	207	119		
N / R	-/-	25/18+2	-/-	-/0	-/-	20/15	-/-	-/0	-/-	-/-
grams CHO / Exercise (min)	-/-	40/-	20/-	72/-	-/-	118/-	-/45	-/-	-/-	-/-
Event1 / Event2	-/-	-/-	-/-	-/-	-/-	-/-	-/-	-/-	-/-	-/-
Comments										

Figure 7.1 Enhanced logbook (courtesy of Mellitus Manager® by MetaMedix, Inc.)

Chart (Graphic) Options

A pie chart is one of the easiest charts to create. You select the pie option from your program menu after downloading data from the meter. Suppose you want to know how often during the day your blood sugars are above or below your target range. The pie chart will appear with three shaded areas. Grey may represent the number of readings within the target range. Let's say black represents the readings above that range and white represents readings below that range. You can see in Figure 7.2 how easy it is to see the balance of normal to abnormal blood sugar.

Or, you could create a pie chart showing the average of breakfast readings or bedtime readings, and so forth. Your pie could represent a day, a week or a month. You can use colors or patterns instead of black and white.

A bar chart can easily make comparisons of various data. Suppose you want to know how much your blood sugar rises or falls after a meal. A simple bar chart will show you average readings before and after breakfast, lunch and dinner. You can add other times of day as well. If the "before" and "after" bars are much too high or much too low, you can quickly determine if you should change your diet or your insulin doses. See Figure 7.3.

Either the pie or the bar chart

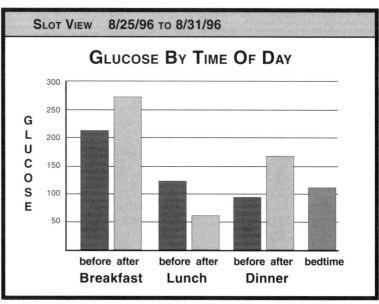

Figure 7.3 A Sample Bar Chart

can be as simple or as complex as you like. If you want to see more or less information, it's easy to edit your chart with most programs.

A line graph was used in the Smart Charts in the last chapter. It can clearly show the pattern of sugar highs and lows in a typical day or week. In that example, the vertical left line of the graph represents glucose in either mg/dl or mmol. The bottom horizontal line represents the date or time of day a reading was recorded. A gray horizontal bar, or two horizontal lines could represent your target range.

Each reading is indicated by a dot at the intersection of the glucose and time coordinates. The dots are connected by a line. The graph makes it clear when and how often your blood sugars rise above or fall below your target range.

Perhaps you want to compare how well you do with different types of insulins or on different diets. On a line graph, one line could represent diet one, one line is diet two and a third line is diet three. By comparing each for a week, you can easily see which one is doing a better job of keeping your blood sugars normal.

A scatter chart superimposes several days' readings, with each reading represented by a dot, on a single 24 hour day. These charts are often called a standard day or modal day, and give an overall impression of blood sugar trends by time of day. It also allows you to see at a glance when you are testing (or not testing).

The great thing about computer charting is that the computer can be told to do as much work as you like. The same basic data can appear in all kinds of graphic displays. Why not create your own custom styles?

FINDING TRENDS AND PATTERNS

As you create your charts, you will soon notice some common patterns. Perhaps most of your lows occur in the afternoon. Perhaps you wake up with high sugars. Or, your chart shows that you are experiencing more lows than you realized. It is important to find these trends so that you can better manage your overall diabetes care.

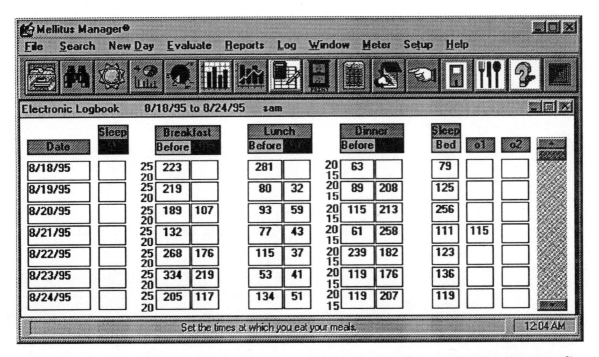

Figure 7.4 A Sample Blood Sugar Software Program (courtesy of Mellitus Manager®)

Your computer can produce a summary report that includes all relevant data on readings, insulin doses, events, etc. This summary, usually one or two pages, is a condensed report of your overall diabetes control. Since optimal presentation is the goal for a summary, you will find this report extremely useful when visiting your physician.

The summary will probably provide a line graph of a standard day and pie graphs showing mealtime readings within and outside your target range. A combination line graph might show the period since your last appointment, or the past 14 days. A statistics report could list all relevant glucose readings. And so on.

WORKING WITH YOUR HEALTH CARE TEAM

Presenting accurate, detailed data on your blood sugar control will help your physician, and others such as dieticians and diabetes educators, to evaluate your progress. Trouble spots and important trends will be obvious. The computer chart data can help you and your health care team make more informed decisions regarding your diabetes care.

SUMMARY

For computer users, a relatively small investment can mean better information through better record keeping. Downloading data from a glucose meter directly to a computer software program is a great time-saver and ensures a high degree of accuracy in reporting.

Data can be presented in different forms, from a simple logbook to more elaborate charts. The charts make it easy to spot trends and trouble spots. A summary report created by computer will be invaluable to your health care team in helping you better manage your diabetes care.

Better charting through computers is the first step towards a more comprehensive system for improving your care. As the products become more sophisticated, keeping track of your blood sugar could be as easy as logging on.

A World Of Online Resources For Diabetes

Internet

Browse:　　http://www.diabetesnet.com (to view *Mellitus Manager*® and other
　　　　　　　information and products by and for people with diabetes)
　　　　　http://www.castleweb.com
　　　　　http://www.diabetes.org
　　　　　http://nhic-nt.health.org
　　　　　http://www.niddk.nih.gov
　　　　　http://www.tyrell.net/~diabetes
　　　　　http://www1.infowest.com/doctor
　　　　　http://www.nd.edu/~hhowisen/diabetes.html
　　　　　http://www.demon.co.uk/diabetic/index.html
　　　　　http://www.biostat.wisc.edu/diaknow/index.htm
　　　　　http://freenet.carleton.ca/freeport/social.services/diabetes/menu
　　　　　http://www.cis.ohio-state.edu/hypertext/faq/usenet/diabetes/top.html

Mailing Lists:　email "subscribe diabetic firstname lastname" to listserv@lehigh.edu
　　　　　　　with no other information. To unsubscribe send only "signoff diabetic"
　　　　　email "subscribe type_one name@address" to listserv@netcom.com. To
　　　　　　　unsubscribe, send "unsubscribe type_one name@address"
　　　　　email "subscribe diabetes-news" to listserv@netcom.com To unsubscribe,
　　　　　　　send "unsubscribe diabetes-news"

Newsgroups:　misc.health.diabetes
　　　　　　alt.support.diabetes.kids

Search:　　http://www.yahoo.com
　　　　　http://www2.infoseek.com
　　　　　http://lycos.cs.cmu.edu
　　　　　http://webcrawler.com

Bulletin Boards:

Black Bag BBS in Collegeville, PA	(610) 454-7396
Diabetes Discussion BBS in Austin, TX	(512) 451-9737
Cracker Barrel BBS in Falmouth, VA	(703) 899-2285
Guilde of High Sorcery BBS in San Diego, CA	(619) 575-8249

Commercial On-Line Companies

Compuserve　　(800) 524-3388　When online, type GO DIABETES
America Online　(800) 827-6364　GO to Lifestyles and Interests, then Better
　　　　　　　　　Health and Fitness, then message center, then Self-help
　　　　　　　　　and Support Groups
Prodigy　　　　(800) 776-3449　Medical support BB, then choose Diabetes

Eternity is a terrible thought.
I mean where is it going to end.

Tom Stoppard

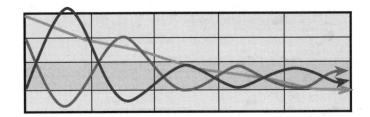

CARB COUNTING—YOUR KEY TO NUTRITION CONTROL

8

Those who use flexible insulin therapy want a meal planning approach that's as exact and as flexible as their injections. *Counting the grams of carbohydrate in foods* offers the most precise and flexible approach available. It gives more exacting control than the traditional exchange system, and in many ways it's easier to learn and use.

This chapter describes:

- Why you want to count carbohydrates
- How carbohydrates affect insulin need
- How to calculate your daily need for carbohydrate
- Which foods have carbohydrate and how to count them
- How to create a healthy meal plan based on carb counting
- Plus the "bigger picture" in healthy eating

The exchange system which many people use is based on estimates of the average nutrient values for each of six classes of foods: breads, fruits, vegetables, milk, fats, and meat (or protein). This generalized diet approach is an excellent way to provide balance in nutrient intake. But it is a less exact way to measure the number of grams of carbohydrate in food. For someone already using the exchange system, this imprecision can be overlooked if the blood sugars are well controlled.

Carb counting has advantages for control because the primary factor in food that affects blood sugars is carbohydrate. The grams of carbohydrate contained in the foods in a meal are calculated and added together. Then the total grams are balanced with a matching dose of Regular taken 30 to 45 minutes before the meal. Regular taken to cover the carbohydrate is approximately half the insulin a person takes all day. So carb counting provides the user with a very precise way to manage this important part of controlling their blood sugar. It does not replace, however, the other primary goal of eating a wide variety of healthy foods each day.

WHY COUNT CARBS?

Carb counting directly measures how high a meal will drive the blood sugar. This allows food to be precisely balanced with Carb Regular or with exercise. Better control is the outcome when you know how many grams of carbohydrate is in the foods you eat, and how many units of Regular or the amount of exercise needed to balance them.

Food is made up of three fuels that affect the blood sugar: carbohydrate, fat and protein. Carbohydrates by far have the largest impact on the blood sugar. Because carbohydrates are so important, the Regular insulin given for a meal or snack is calculated to match the food's carbohydrate content or "count". Carb counting is the most accurate way to determine the dose of Regular to give for each meal. (Any system that quantifies food, estimates insulin need, and achieves good blood sugar control can be used as long as it works!) The only carbs not covered with insulin are those that are being used to balance exercise or to raise a low blood sugar.

Some 90 to 100 percent of the calories from digestible carbohydrates (starches and sugars) end up as glucose. This glucose rapidly starts to raise the blood sugar following a meal. This means that the amount of insulin needed to cover a meal or snack can be closely estimated by simply counting the grams of carbohydrate contained in the meal.

To measure the impact that a meal will have on the blood sugar, either the exchange system, counting calories, or the TAG (total available glucose) system can be used. If one of these systems, or even your own intuition, is working well for you, don't change a thing. But if your control is not what you desire, or you're interested in a more flexible, logical, and exact approach to blood sugar control, learn carb counting.

WHAT ELSE AFFECTS THE BLOOD SUGAR?

Food contains energy in the form of carbohydrate, fat, and protein, plus many other important metabolic helpers like vitamins and minerals. All foods, except pure alcohol, contribute glucose to the bloodstream. But the contributions are not equal. Fats have almost no direct affect on blood sugars over the short run. Only when an excess of certain fats are eaten can they block insulin action, making blood sugars rise more than expected after some high fat meals. Foods which are high in fat do have a negative impact on health, however, since they can lead to *obesity, heart disease, and higher blood sugars.*

Fat in the diet can also affect blood sugar control. On the one hand, fat delays the intestinal absorption of carbohydrate and can reduce the ex-

---

Today's Eating Guidelines:

1. Eat a variety of healthy, nutritious foods,
2. Reduce fat and protein to reasonable amounts,
3. Then balance your carbohydrate with insulin and exercise.

---

pected rise in blood sugars after a meal.[21] Ice cream, which has a low glycemic index (less likely to raise the blood sugar), is a good example of this. On the other hand, high fat meals may create resistance to insulin for eight to 16 hours after a meal and make the blood sugar rise.[22, 23] Pizza is a good example of this.

Excess fat in the diet also appears to be a significant cause of Type II diabetes.[24] Eating a high fat diet over time leads to weight gain and insulin resistance, particularly in those prone to an apple figure or male pattern obesity.[25, 26] Insulin resistance involves changes in metabolism that makes it harder for sugar to be used as fuel, while at the same time extra fat and sugar are being produced and released into the bloodstream. The excess weight and insulin resistance that result are not good for health, and are a major reason the American Heart Association and the American Diabetes Association have recommended less fat and calories in the diet. Most effects of a high fat diet are seen over the long run. Although the effect of fat on blood sugars following a particular high fat meal or snack are usually small,[27] fat, especially saturated and hydrogenated fat, should be reduced in the diet for better health.

The small portions of protein eaten in the diet have a minimal impact.[28] Around half of protein eaten ends up as blood sugar, but the glucose from protein breakdown appears slowly in the blood over several hours following a meal. Because protein makes up only 10 to 20 percent of calories in most people's diet, it determines less than a tenth of the total blood sugar control.

Consuming average amounts of protein usually has little effect on blood sugars. Large quantities of protein, however, can impact the blood sugar because 50 percent of protein calories are slowly converted to glucose over a period of several hours. If an eight-ounce steak or several ounces of cheese are eaten, this can raise blood sugars taken four to 12 hours later.

Following a high-protein dinner, for instance, blood sugars will rise gradually over several hours and reach a peak the following morning. Taking extra Regular for a high protein meal is not recommended because of the slow onset and long duration of this protein effect. A small increase in the evening long-acting insulin can be considered following some high protein meals, but only if there is a consistent pattern where that meal has been shown to raise the next morning's blood sugar. A better plan for blood sugar control (and better protection for the kidneys) is to avoid eating this much protein.

Where's The Carbohydrate?

Healthy diets contain 50 percent to 60 percent of the day's total calories as carbohydrate. (The one exception comes in pregnancy when a 40 percent carbohydrate diet is recommended because blood sugar control is so critical.

Carbohydrate comes from:

- Grains (breads, pasta, cereals)
- Fruits
- Vegetables
- Root crops (potatoes, sweet potatoes, and yams)
- Beer and wine
- Desserts and candies
- Most milk products, except cheese
- **-ose** foods, like sucrose, fructose, maltose

And though you might not eat them often, remember the high carbohydrate content of "splurge" foods like ice cream, cake, pie and candy. With carbohydrate counting, you can learn to handle occasional splurges so that they don't destroy your hard-won diabetes control.

What Are Grams?

A gram is a unit of weight like pounds or ounces. Because of its very small size (it takes 28 grams to make a single ounce), grams can be used to accurately measure carbohydrate. Unfortunately, simply weighing a food does not tell how much carbohydrate it has. For example, a cup of milk weighs 224 grams, two graham cracker squares weigh 14 grams, and a tablespoon of sugar weighs 12 grams. But all contain the same amount of carbohydrate: 12 grams. (The milk contains water and the graham crackers contain fiber and other ingredients that are not carbohydrate.) Although their total weights are different, these three food items will require the same dose of Carb Regular to cover them because they each have 12 grams of carbohydrate.

How Many Carbs Do You Need In A Day?

Your daily carbohydrate goal is based on how many total calories you need. A healthy diet gets most of its calories, normally 50 to 65 percent, from carbohydrates. A person who needs 2000 calories a day would get 1000 to 1300 of those calories from the carbohydrate in breads, grains, vegetables, fruits, low-fat milk, and so on. Since there are four calories in each gram of carbohydrate, a person eating 2000 calories per day would need between 250 to 325 grams (between 1000 calories divided by four and 1300 calories divided by four) of carbohydrate.

That number becomes the basis of a carb counting meal plan. The total amount of carbohydrate for the day is divided up among the meals and snacks a person normally eats.

Remember, if you use a good multiple injection regimen, snacks are not as necessary. Once the background insulin has been correctly set, you now have the freedom to enjoy snacks and cover them with an injection of Regular when you want, not when the insulin says you must.

Healthy Carbohydrates

In a healthy diet most of these carbohydrates will come from nutrient-dense foods like whole grains, fruits, legumes, vegetables, and nonfat or lowfat milk and yogurt. Nutrient-dense foods are ones that have a high volume of nutrients like vitamins, minerals, fiber and protein for their calorie content. Less healthy carbohydrates are contained in low nutrient foods such as candy and regular sodas. They lack the other nutrients that your cells require to remain healthy. Furthermore, they can cause blood sugar spiking. The carbohydrates and nutrients found in nutrient-dense foods like brown rice and broccoli give you the most health value per calorie, as well as the best blood sugars.

> ### "Lente" Carbohydrates
>
> Just like long-acting insulins, there are long-acting carbs. Useful at bedtime and during longer exercise, these foods keep the blood sugar from falling over longer periods of time.
>
> Examples are beans (lima, pinto, etc.), green apples, PowerBars, raw cornstarch, pasta al dente, barley, cracked wheat, parboiled long grain and whole grain rice, and whole rye bread.

THE RIGHT CARB LEVEL FOR YOU

A diet containing 50 to 60 percent of the total calories as carbohydrate is the current recommendation for health. Most people in the United States eat about 40 percent of their calories as carbohydrate, 40 percent as fat, and 20 percent as protein. If you have been eating less than the recommended 50 percent of calories as carbohydrate, you may have difficulty consuming this much carbohydrate at first.

One way to judge whether eating more carbohydrate will be difficult is to simply eat your usual meals for a few days, and keep a record of how much carbohydrate you actually take in. If you find that you are eating significantly less carbohydrate than that recommended in the worksheet on the next page, try increasing your carbohydrate intake by 10 percent while reducing fat and protein calories by the same amount. Because carbohydrate plays such a major role in setting your insulin doses, it is best not to make an abrupt change in how much carbohydrate you eat.

Some people find that they can achieve blood sugar control more easily and also reduce their risk of hypoglycemia (because they are also on smaller doses of Regular) when they eat less carbohydrate in their meals. The reason a higher carbohydrate intake is recommended is that this reduces calories coming from fat and protein in the diet. A reduced fat and protein intake lessens risks for heart disease and kidney disease respectively, risks which are quite high in people with diabetes. Over 70 percent of people with Type II diabetes, for instance, die as a result of cardiovascular disease, while some 30 percent of those with Type I diabetes die directly or indirectly from kidney disease.

If your blood sugar control is worse when you eat more calories from carbohydrate, the poor control may offset any benefit obtained through an "improved" diet. If you find you have a problem balancing your carbs with Regular, discuss how to better balance Regular and carbohydrates with your physician or dietician.

Your total daily carbohydrate allowance (either the amount calculated above or a lower value based on your current intake) can be divided into the amounts that you prefer for each meal or snack. Table 8.3 shows three examples of how 225 grams of total daily carbohydrate can be divided among meals and snacks. Your own pattern can be based on your personal preferences and needs.

DAILY CARBS WORKSHEET

Fill in the blanks to determine how many grams of carbohydrate you need each day. We encourage you to consult with your dietician for specific help.

1. Determine your *desired weight* in pounds. See Table 8.1.

    My weight goal equals _____ lbs. (If you are overweight, a 10 percent loss is ideal.)

2. Choose a *calorie factor* that best describes your activity level. Table 8.2 gives you calorie factors for different levels of activity.

    My calorie factor from Table 8.2 equals _____

3. Determine your *total daily calorie need*:

    ___*140*___ lbs. multiplied by ___*13*___ equals ___*1820*___ calories

    my desired weight   **my calorie factor**   **number of calories I need each day**

4. Divide your total daily calories by 8 (1/2 of calories as carbohydrate and 1/4 gram per calorie) to determine how many *total grams of carbohydrate you need each day* when you eat a 50 percent carbohydrate diet:

    ___*1820*___ calories divided by 8 equals ___*227*___ grams

    calories/day   **grams of carbohydrate/day**

5. Now decide how you want to *split up* these total carbohydrates for the day into different meals:

breakfast	_____ grams
AM snack	_____ grams
lunch	_____ grams
PM snack	_____ grams
dinner	_____ grams
eve. snack	_____ grams

Table 8.1 Optimum weights for men and women of any age:

Height	Weight in pounds
4' 10"	91-119
4' 11"	94-124
5' 0"	97-128
5' 1"	101-132
5' 2"	104-137
5" 3"	107-141
5" 4"	111-146
5' 5"	114-150
5' 6"	118-155
5" 7"	121-160
5' 8"	125-164
5' 9'	129-169
5" 10"	132-174
5" 11"	136-179
6' 0"	140-184

Table 8.2 Calorie Factors For Different Levels Of Activity

Activity Level	Calorie Factor Male	Female
Very Sedentary: Limited activity; slow walking; mostly sitting.	13	11.5
Sedentary: Recreational activities include walking; bowling, fishing, or similar activities.	14	12.5
Moderately Active: Recreational activities include 18 hole golf, aerobic dancing, pleasure swimming, etc.	15	13.5
Active: Greater than 20 minutes of jogging, swimming, competitive tennis or similar activities more than three times per week.	16	14.5
Super Active: At least one hour of vigorous activity such as football, weight training, or full-court basketball four or more days per week.	17	15.5

FINDING THE CARBOHYDRATE CONTENT OF FOODS

To count carbohydrates, you'll need information on the carbohydrate content of foods. You will find this information in Appendix A in the back of the book. You can also refer to nutrition labels, food composition books, or food exchange lists.

Like any new skill, counting grams of carbohydrate will take a couple of weeks for you to master. You'll need to weigh and measure foods consistently. As time passes, you'll have trained your eye to accurately estimate serving sizes and weights, especially when eating out.

Eventually, you'll be able to look at a piece of fruit, a plate of pasta or a combination plate in your favorite restaurant and quickly esti-

Ways To Divide Carbs Through The Day			
Example 1: Big breakfast & lunch, light dinner & bedtime snack			
Example 2: Light breakfast and frequent snacks			
Example 3: Carbs evenly divided among meals			
Meal or Snack	**Example 1**	**Example 2**	**Example 3**
Breakfast	75 grams	30 grams	75 grams
Morning snack		15 grams	
Lunch	70 grams	45 grams	75 grams
Afternoon snack		30 grams	
Dinner	40 grams	75 grams	75 grams
Bedtime snack	40 grams	30 grams	

Table 8.3 There Are Many Ways to Split The Day's Carbs

mate its carbohydrate count accurately, without weighing, measuring or looking up a thing. This, of course, is easier if you tend to eat the same thing often, as many people do. Be patient but persistent as you develop this skill. When you can precisely adjust your Carb Regular to match the carbohydrates you eat, it will be worth all the effort.

WHAT EQUIPMENT DO I NEED

To measure carbohydrates, you will need measuring equipment, such as a digital gram scale, measuring spoons and cup. Measuring cups and spoons measure volume. Scales measure weight. For some foods there is a big difference. For example 10 ounces of Cheerios® *by volume* (1 ¼ cups) is equal to one ounce *by weight* (28 grams). Be sure you're clear on whether measures are for volume or weight. Many nutrition labels and food composition tables give both types of measure.

Measuring Cups and Spoons: Accurate measuring cups and spoons are available in many different places and price ranges. Use a glass measuring container that allows you to "sight" across the top of liquids and a measuring cup that lets you scrape a knife across the top to get the exact measure for dry items such as cereal and rice.

Gram scales: A gram scale is the best way to measure the actual weight of a food in grams. A good scale will weigh food accurately within one or two grams. Look also for a tare feature that allows you to zero out the weight of containers. This lets you pour your food directly into the serving bowl, and eliminates the hassle of weighing foods on the scale and then moving them into your bowl.

If you can afford a few extra dollars, a computerized gram scale can save you a great deal of effort. These scales are pre-programmed with information about how much carbohydrate is contained in different foods. When you enter the name of a food and place it on the scale, the scale automatically calculates the grams of carbohydrate in the food being weighed.

Several brands of scales are available, ranging in price from $50 to $80 for digital scales to almost $200 for a scale which contains an internal database of foods. Scales can be found in gourmet and kitchen shops. Mail order suppliers, like Nasco (901 Janesville Ave.; Fort Atkinson, Wis. 53538; 1-800-558-9595) or the Diabetic Reader (1-800-735-7726) have gram scales for sale.

Using Food Labels

All packaged foods today have a "Nutrition Facts" label on them. This label contains information about the nutrition contained in that product, including the numbers of calories, carbohydrate, protein, and fat contained in *one serving*. These labels are great for carb counting because they give the exact number of grams of carbohydrate contained in a serving. An example is given on the right.

If you're eating a food that has all the information you need on the label, you can calculate insulin coverage easily. For example, an 8 ounce carton of Elsie's Lowfat Yogurt has a label that tells you that an 8 ounce serving has 43 grams of carbohydrate. Armed with this information and knowing how many grams of carbohydrate are covered by one unit of insulin from Chapter 10, you can figure out how much Carb Regular is needed to cover this food. If the serving you eat is different from the serving size listed on the package, you will have to weigh or measure your actual serving and do some calculations.

Carb Counting And The 450 Rule

A useful tool for carb counting is the 450 Rule. This rule applies only to people with Type I diabetes using flexible insulin therapy. The rule estimates how many grams of carbohydrate will be covered by one unit of Regular insulin. The 450 Rule says that the number of grams of carbohydrate covered by one unit of Regular equals 450 divided by the total daily insulin dose.

For example, someone on 50 units of insulin a day will need a unit of Regular for every nine grams of carbohydrate (450/50 = 9). If they have three slices of bread (15 grams each), they should be able to cover this 45 grams with five units of Regular. (ONLY if on flexible insulin therapy.)

THE 450 RULE	What Is Your Total Daily Insulin Dose?	Grams of Carb One Unit of Regular is Likely To Cover:
	20 units	22 grams
	25 units	18 grams
	30 units	15 grams
	40 units	11 grams
	50 units	9 grams
	60 units	8 grams
	75 units	6 grams
	100 units	5 grams

Table 8.4 How to determine carb coverage from your total daily insulin dose

Advantage: Very easy. Requires reading labels.

What you need: Food labels, measuring cup.

How: Food labels contain all the information needed to do carb counting. Just be sure your serving is the *same size as the serving on the label.*

Example: Two servings of Creamy Wild Rice

1. Look at Fig. 8.5. Let's say you want to eat a cup of Uncle Bob's Wild Rice, but a serving size is a half cup.

2. Look on the label for the number of carbohydrates in one serving (a ½ cup).

Nutrition Facts:	
Uncle Bob's Creamy Wild Rice	
Serving Size	1/2 cup cooked
Serv. Per Cont.	1
Calories	130
Protein	4 grams
Total Carb.	23 grams
Total Fat	1 grams

Fig. 8.5 Sample food label

3. Multiply this number (23 grams) by two to determine the carbohydrate you will be eating:

    Carbs in a half cup portion   =   23 grams
    Multiply by 2 for your one cup serving   =   X   2
                                                           46 grams of carbohydrate

4. You will be eating 46 grams of carbohydrate.

Using Food Exchange Lists

Food exchange lists can be used to *approximate* the carbohydrate content of foods. In some cases, the exchange system will not accurately describe your particular food. Here are two examples that show instances in which using exchanges to estimate carbohydrate might have different results:

| **Example 1:** | A slice of Wonder bread (1 bread exchange) | = | 15 grams of carb |
| | Actual carb value | = | **15 grams of carb** |

Here the values are the same, so there's no problem.

| **Example 2:** | A slice of Lieken bread (1 bread exchange) | = | 15 grams of carb |
| | Actual carb value of Lieken bread | = | **29 grams of carb** |

Here the actual carb value is nearly twice the exchange value. With most food items, the differences between the exchange system value and the actual grams of carbohydrate won't be this large. But when estimating your dose of Carb Regular, if the carbohydrate content of several items in a meal is estimated using exchanges, these differences may be large enough to cause control problems.

Using Nutrition Books and Cookbooks

Food composition books and brochures, just like nutrition labels, describe the amount of carbohydrate in a typical serving size of each food. You will need to weigh or measure your actual serving, and then do the necessary calculations to learn how many grams of carbohydrate are contained in your own serving.

Advantage: Many cookbooks have the carbohydrate content and exchanges listed with each recipe. These are great for counting carbohydrates while preparing meals at home, as long as you measure the number of servings you eat.

What you need: Books; measuring tools to determine serving size.

How: Look for books in the "Nutrition and Diet" section of your local bookstore or library. Look also for recipes with carbohydrate content in the "Food" section of your local newspaper.

- *Calories and Carbohydrates* by Barbara Kraus (Penguin Books, New York)—lists 8,000 foods
- *The Carbohydrate Gram Counter* by Corinne Netzer (Dell, New York)—lists 10,000 foods
- *Food Values* by Jean Pennington, Ph.D., R.D. (Harper Collins Publishers, New York) —comprehensive, includes many vitamins and minerals
- *Total Nutrition Guide* by Jean Carper (Bantam Books, New York)—comprehensive: carbs, fats, minerals, fast foods

These two books are great for looking up many brand name foods and for eating out:
- *Convenience Food Facts* by Arlene Monk (DCI/ChroniMed, $10.95) gives the grams of carbohydrate in 1,500 popular brand name products
- *Restaurant Companion* by Hope Warshaw (Surrey Books, $9.95) If you eat out often in restaurants, this will be a big help. Many restaurants also have their own brochures that describe the nutritional content of menu items

For information on a vegetarian diet using the exchange system, the book below helps:
- *The Healing Power of Foods Cookbook* by Michael T. Murray, N.D. (Prima Publishing)

Using a Gram Scale

A few foods like table sugar and lollipops are entirely carbohydrate. When placed on a gram scale, their weight tells you immediately how many grams of carbohydrate they contain. But most foods have only part of their total weight as carbohydrate. The carbohydrate content of these foods can be determined by weighing them and then multiplying this total weight by a "carb factor" which gives the percentage of the food's total weight that is actually carbohydrate.

For instance, when you eat a food like fruit that has no label—and you don't have a computerized scale that does the work for you—you have to calculate the grams of carbohydrate in your serving. Different calculation methods will be useful under different circumstances or with different foods.

Advantage: Convenient for measuring carbs in odd-sized foods like fruits, unsliced bread, cereals, or casseroles.

What you need:
1. A gram scale
2. A calculator
3. A list of Carb Factors like those in Appendix A at the back of this book.

How: To find the amount of carbohydrate a particular food has:
1. Weigh the food on a gram scale to find its total weight in grams.
2. Find that food's Carb Factor in one of the Food Groups listed in Appendix A.
3. Multiply the food's total weight in grams by its Carb Factor.
4. This number is the number of grams of carbohydrate you are eating.

Example: Six ounces of cooked spaghetti—to find the amount of carbohydrate:
1. After zeroing out your plate on a scale, you place the amount of cooked spaghetti you want to eat onto it. You find the portion you want weighs 200 grams on the scale.
2. In Appendix A, you find that cooked plain spaghetti has a carbohydrate factor of 0.26 or 26 percent carbohydrate by weight.
3. Multiply the spaghetti's total weight in grams by its Carb Factor.

Weight of spaghetti portion	=	200 grams
Carbohydrate factor for spaghetti	=	X 0.26
		52 grams of carbohydrate

4. So, when you eat 200 grams of spaghetti by weight, you'll eat 52 grams of carbohydrate.

Example: A slice of French bread—to find the amount of carbohydrate:
1. Slice a piece of bread from the loaf and place it on your gram scale. You find that it weights 80 grams.
2. In Appendix A you find that the Carb Factor for bread equals 0.50 (This means that 50 percent or half the total weight of bread is carbohydrate.).
3. Multiply its weight (80 grams) by 0.50 to determine the carbohydrate:
   80 grams of French bread times 0.50 equals 40 grams of carbohydrate
4. There are 40 grams of carbohydrate in this slice of French bread.

CARB COUNTING IS NOT THE ONLY WAY

There are other ways to improve your control with food. Many people use the exchange system where foods are divided into broad categories like breads, meats, and fruits, and then portions are provided that have about the same nutritional value. For categories like bread, fruit, and vegetables, this value is largely the food's carbohydrate content. Other people eyeball their meals and estimate portions by their size on a plate or the glass or bowl it fits into.

Let's look at how three busy men handled a meal problem. One morning all three men came into the office of Creative Carol, R.D., the nutritionist. Each complained that he woke up in the morning with great blood sugars, but after the "very same breakfast that I always eat" and the same dose of insulin, the blood sugar at lunch would always vary.

After questioning each about nighttime reactions and activity, Carol suspected that the amount of carbohydrate for breakfast was not really the same. So she worked with each to find an appropriate solution.

They all liked having the same brand of cereal with fruit, a glass of milk, a glass of tomato juice, plus a slice of cheese for breakfast. Over the following week after their appointment with Carol, each tracked his blood sugar and found the readings had indeed improved. To see what each one did after getting home, see Table 8.6.

Note that one of these gentlemen, Mike, even uses "eyeballing" to measure his foods. This can work, but only if you are skillful at it. For instance, Mike usually eats out at the same three restaurants and has two favorite meals on each menu. At his Italian restaurant, he likes linguine with clear pesto sauce and clams, a house salad, and splits a piece of apple pie with his wife. By tracking his readings for a few weeks, he found that 7 units of Regular works great for this meal.

WEIGHT GAIN

Many horror stories abound about people gaining weight when they begin to control their blood sugars. This does not have to happen. The road to true blood sugar control lies in eating what you need and then adjusting your insulin to handle that amount of food.

When your blood sugar is in good control, your body behaves just like it did before you had diabetes. If you eat too much, you gain weight. If you eat less, you lose weight.

Keep track of your weight and your appetite. These tell you whether you're actually eating the right amount of food. Keep the fat and protein calories at moderate levels, and adjust your insulin to match an appropriate carbohydrate intake. And stay very active and involved in your life!

THE BIGGER NUTRITION PICTURE

When you have mastered the art of carbohydrate counting, you will be an expert in how to balance your insulin and food intake to achieve blood sugar control. As important as it is, however, blood sugar control is not the only health goal you have while eating. Your overall health is dependent on eating a wide variety of nutrient-rich foods.

When ordering his three or four colossal triple bacon & cheese mega-burgers with jumbo fries, Leon made sure his drink of choice was always 'sugar-free.'

The amount of fat in your diet appears to be very important to health. High intake of fat has been associated with greater risk for heart disease, cancer and obesity. These health problems are even more important to people with diabetes than they are to others. Heart disease is twice as common in people who have diabetes as it is in the general population. Because of this extra cardiac risk, a fat intake of no more than 20 percent to 30 percent of total calories is recommended by the American Diabetes Association, the American Heart Association, and the American Dietetic Association. This focus on reducing

Matt	Tom	Mike
Matt uses Carb Counting:	Tom uses the exchange system:	Mike eyeballs his entire diet:
Brand X Cereal: 45 grams 1/2 banana: 15 grams 1 cup milk: 12 grams 6 oz. tomato juice: 8 grams 1 oz. cheese: 0 grams	Brand X Cereal: 3 breads 1/2 banana: 1 fruit 1 cup milk: 1 milk 6 oz. tomato juice: ½ fruit 1 oz. cheese: 1 protein	Brand X Cereal always in the same bowl, with 1/2 banana, milk in the same glass, tomato juice in the same glass, plus 1 slice of packaged cheese.

Table 8.6 Three ways to approach the diet for control

fat intake may be one reason for the gradual reduction in the number of heart attacks over the last few years.

Most people cut back by cutting down on fats added to foods (butter, margarine, sour cream, salad dressings, oils and shortening used for frying, etc.). They also choose protein foods that are lower in fat or that contain better types of fat (fish, skinless chicken, nonfat milk, and nonfat cheese products, for example). Diets that are lower in animal protein have also been shown to slow the development and progression of diabetic kidney disease. Thirty to 35 percent of people with Type I diabetes will develop kidney disease, so keeping meat portions smaller is highly recommended.

After talking about reducing our intake of greasy old favorites, it seems only fair to talk about a change in the diabetes diet that is good news. As most of us remember, the dietary harangue in the past was "No Sugar!" That taboo has been loosening in recent years as blood sugar testing has shown that it's possible to retain glycemic control when eating some "splurge foods" if we know how to account for their sometimes hefty carbohydrate content.

Sugar is no longer banned from coffee, nor jelly from toast, nor an occasional small piece of pie from the dinner table. It appears that it may, in fact, be healthier to have a small amount of applebutter (which has some sugar but no fat in it) on your waffle, rather than the butter or margarine that were recommended in the past.

No one really benefits nutritionally from an excess of these high-calorie, low-nutrient foods, whether or not he or she has diabetes. However, small amounts of sweets can add flavor to a diet and, if chosen wisely, make avoiding fatty foods a little easier. Be careful though: sugar almost always travels with fat. For instance, a chocolate candy bar gets about 60 percent of its calories from fat!

Whether you include some sweets in your meals or not, the key to blood sugar control is to determine the amount of carbohydrate in your food and cover it with an appropriate amount of insulin. This, together with a nutrient rich, low fat, low protein diet, are vital parts of a healthy lifestyle for those with diabetes and those without.

The waist is a terrible thing to mind.
Ziggy (Tom Wilson)

WHAT YOU NEED TO KNOW ABOUT INSULIN

CHAPTER 9.   TYPES OF INSULIN AND HOW THEY ARE USED

CHAPTER 10.   TIPS ON INSULIN DOSES AND ORAL AGENTS
IN TYPE II DIABETES

CHAPTER 11.   TIPS ON INSULIN

CHAPTER 12.   SEVERE HIGH BLOOD SUGARS AND KETOACIDOSIS

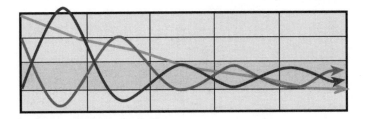

TYPES OF INSULIN AND HOW THEY ARE USED

9

To recap briefly, in past chapters you have learned about:

- How flexible insulin therapy works
- The importance of normal blood sugars
- How to use various charting methods to find blood sugar patterns
- The importance of carb counting to control

With this knowledge you can better take control of your blood sugars. In this chapter you will learn:

- The role of insulin in blood sugar control
- Why different long-acting insulins are used
- How to use Regular to cover carbohydrates
- How to use Regular to cover high blood sugars

THE ROLE OF NATURAL INSULIN

Natural insulin controls glucose entry into some cells, helps regulate production and release of fats as fuel, and helps certain amino acids that create enzymes and structural proteins to enter cells. Beta cells in a normal pancreas deliver precise amounts of insulin into the blood to move glucose from the blood into fat, muscle and liver cells. At the same time, enough glucose remains in the blood so the brain and nervous system receive the fuel they depend on for their vital functions. Part of this balancing act comes from the release of other hormones like epinephrine, growth hormone and cortisol. These other hormones counterbalance insulin by releasing glucose at the appropriate time from glycogen stores within the liver and muscles.

Since the body needs fuel all the time, insulin is always present in the bloodstream. When the pancreas is functioning normally, it delivers insulin in two ways to cover two needs:

1. As a constant release (about half the total) to maintain ongoing metabolism;

2. In short spurts (the other half) delivered to cover the carbohydrate in food.

Other things can change the need for insulin, such as an infection (need more insulin) or exercise (need less insulin), but the two needs listed above are key to understanding the use of insulin.

Figure 9.1 shows the normal release of insulin into the blood over a 24-hour period. The shaded area in the figure represents the constant release of background insulin. Following meals, a release of "first phase" insulin is seen. This fast release occurs in the first 15 minutes after eating and

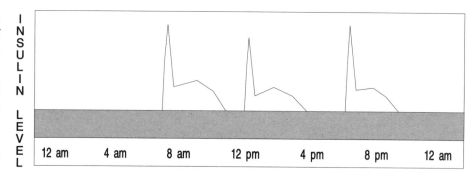

Figure 9.1 Normal Blood Insulin Levels: Background insulin in grey plus after-meal spikes.

comes from insulin waiting in storage areas of the beta cells. This is followed by a more gradual second phase over the next hour and a half to three hours as insulin production gears up in the beta cells. The sharp spikes of insulin above the background level in Figure 9.1 represent first phase insulin release, followed by smaller, longer second phase release.

In contrast, for someone who has diabetes and injects insulin, flexible insulin therapy helps meet three needs:

1. As a constant release for ongoing metabolism (the long-acting insulin)

2. As coverage for carbohydrate in food (Carb Regular)

3. To lower high blood sugars when they occur (High Blood Sugar Regular)

To match these three needs, two groups of insulin are used. One group includes the faster-acting insulins like Regular and a new insulin called Lispro. The other group includes long-acting insulins like Lente, NPH, and Ultralente. These groups have different action times.

Regular starts working in about 20 minutes and keeps working for five to eight hours after an injection. This insulin was discovered by Banting and Best in 1921, and was first used in humans in 1923. Although Regular is the fastest insulin currently available to cover meals, it has a relatively slow onset and a long action time that make it too slow for most meals that rapidly raise the blood sugar. In many people, an injection of Regular allows the blood sugar to rise sharply after a meal but causes it to drop long after the meal is finished.

This slow reaction time for Regular insulin is worsened by excess weight common in Type IIr diabetes. Excess weight delays the action of insulin, and make blood sugars more likely to rise after meals.

Insulin	Start	Peak	End	Lows most likely at
Lispro	10 m	1.5 h	4 h	2-4 h
Regular	20 m	3-4 h	8 h	3-7 h
NPH	1.5 h	4-10 h	22 h	6-13 h
Lente	2.5 h	6-12 h	24 h	7-14 h
Ultralente	4 h	10-18 h	36 h	10-22 h

Table 9.2 Action Times for Insulins

Lilly has nearly completed testing a new, faster insulin called Lispro, which should be available in 1996. Lispro is genetically modified from Regular into an insulin that works almost twice as fast. It represents a major advance in three ways: it can be taken right before a meal, it keeps post-meal readings from spiking, and it is gone in a little over 3 hours, about the same time as most foods. Lispro also corrects high blood sugars faster.

Long-acting insulins were developed in the 1940s and 50s when Regular was chemically linked to zinc to form Lente and Ultralente, and to a protein called Neutral Protamine Hagedorn to form NPH. These linkages slowed absorption from the injection site to create insulins that work for longer periods of time. Table 9.2 shows the start, peak, and end times for various insulins.

Compared to Regular, long-acting insulins are slower to start working but they last longer. Lente and NPH have no significant impact on the blood sugar for 3 to 4 hours, while Ultralente begins to have an impact in five to six hours. Lente and NPH can last up to 24 hours and Ultralente up to 40 hours.

ADVANTAGE OF FIT

Using flexible insulin therapy, those who produce little or no insulin will inject insulin three or more times a day. Compared to 1 or 2 injections, the great advantage of frequent injections is that each of the three needs for insulin in diabetes can be covered separately. As insulin needs are clearly defined and each need is covered with a particular insulin dose, these doses can be tested to be sure they are doing what you want them to do.

For instance, if someone is having afternoon lows, this may be caused by too much of the morning long-acting insulin or too much Regular for lunch. Using FIT, the person can find out which insulin is causing the problem, by skipping lunch along with their lunch Regular. If the blood sugar falls sharply, the morning long-acting insulin is causing the problem. If it doesn't, the lunch Regular is likely too high.

Flexible insulin therapy lets you judge your need for insulin more easily. That is its greatest advantage. You can determine your own need with testing done over a six-week period (described in the next seven chapters). To briefly summarize this testing, you:

1. Skip meals to check if the long-acting insulin is working properly
2. Learn to count carbohydrates in meals and match them correctly with Regular
3. Learn how much Regular is needed to correct high blood sugars

Most people need to make occasional minor adjustments in their insulin doses. For instance, more insulin is usually required during the winter months of November through February or March. During these months, we are less active and our diets are higher in calories and fat. As spring approaches and activity rises, the need for insulin again drops. The principles you learn in this book will let you make these adjustments at the right time.

MORE ON LONG-ACTING INSULIN

About half of the total daily insulin supply is needed as a steady background insulin flow that controls the three fuels—carbohydrate, fat and protein.[29] Due to variability in how long-acting insulins work and because of the advantage of having an extra cap on the blood sugar, 45 to 60 percent of the total daily insulin dose usually ends up being given as long-acting insulin.

Long-acting insulins work best when given two or three times a day. This minimizes their peaking action, spreading the insulin action more evenly through the day. A morning dose is generally given before breakfast, followed by an evening dose before the evening meal or at bedtime. A third dose may help flatten the insulin delivery. The morning dose is generally larger than the evening to help offset normal food intake during the day. This "capping" effect helps control post-meal blood sugars.

For some people, the evening dose of long-acting insulin may need to be the largest. Extra nighttime insulin helps those with Type I diabetes who have a strong Dawn Phenomenon and many people with Type IIr diabetes who have their highest blood sugars at breakfast. Once the doses of long-acting insulin are set, minor adjustments are needed to balance seasonal changes, changes in weight or activity, or to balance the menstrual cycle.

Note also that because their action begins slowly and lasts 20 to 40 hours, long-acting insulins are *NOT* used to lower random high blood sugars.

Long-acting insulins deliver the background insulin that's needed to control the availability and use of the fuels when you're not eating. *Setting up the long-acting insulin is the most important step in controlling the blood sugar.* Doses of Regular insulin cannot be determined accurately until the doses of long-acting insulin have been correctly set. For instance, if the long-acting insulin is too high, Carb Regular might not be needed to cover a snack or meal, or if Regular is given for a meal, it would be less insulin than expected. With excess background insulin, if the blood sugar were 80 to 120 mg/dl (5 to 6.7 mmol) before a meal and the meal (and Carb Regular) were skipped, a person's blood sugars will begin to go low shortly afterward.

If the background insulin is too low, just the opposite happens. A person would require larger than normal doses of Regular to cover meals. When a meal (and Carb Regular) is skipped, the blood sugar would climb as the hours passed.

Figure 9.3 shows what happens when the long-acting insulin is too low (A), correctly set (B), and too high (C). The blood sugar trends shown in the graph show what happens to the blood sugar over a 24 hour period in which no eating occurs. The dose of long-acting insulin is correctly set when the blood sugar remains fairly level or drops slightly while fasting (see line B in Figure 9.3).

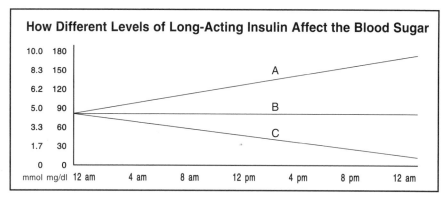

Fig. 9.3 Long-acting insulin: low (A), normal (B), high (C)

MORE ON SHORT-ACTING INSULIN

Once the long-acting insulin dose has been correctly set, Regular insulin serves the other two functions:

1. Carb Regular covers the carbohydrate in meals and snacks

2. High Blood Sugar Regular lowers high blood sugars

Carb Regular

With flexible insulin therapy, Regular insulin (or eventually Lispro) given before each meal mirrors the way a normal pancreas works. The amount of Regular used for each meal is determined by the amount of carbohydrate eaten in that meal. The more carbohydrate eaten, the more Regular used to cover it.

Meal carbohydrates break down rapidly in the digestive tract and start to raise the blood sugar just a few minutes after eating. Compared to the ability of the pancreas to deliver insulin directly into the blood, an injection of Regular into subcutaneous tissue does not start to lower blood sugars until 30 to 90 minutes after it has been given. By giving enough lead time for the Carb Regular to work, the spiking of blood sugars one to two hours after eating is reduced. Regular insulin works best when given at least 30 minutes before a meal when the blood sugar is normal.

However, Carb Regular is *not* used to cover carbohydrates when:

1. Carbohydrate is used to raise a low blood sugar

2. Carbohydrate is used to compensate for extra physical activity

3. You are uncertain about keeping food down due to nausea or vomiting

The correct dose of Regular to carbohydrate for a meal allows the blood sugar to go from 70 to 120 mg/dl (3.9 to 6.7 mmol) before a meal back to 70 to 120 mg/dl (3.9 to 6.7 mmol) four to five hours later.

If your blood sugar is high before a meal and your schedule allows, you will benefit from taking the Carb Regular plus the High Blood Sugar Regular at least 45 to 90 minutes before eating (depending on how high the reading is and how quickly you drop). Post-meal readings can be improved by injecting insulin for the meal and for the high blood sugar, then delaying eating until the blood sugar is below 150 mg/dl (8.3 mmol).

Remember that missing or delaying meals is the most common cause for insulin reactions. *Do not delay eating if you may not be able to later eat the meal for which you've taken insulin.*

High Blood Sugar Regular

Figure 9.4 provides suggestions for how long to delay eating based on how high the blood sugar is and on how fast your blood sugar drops. The three lines in the figure give the time delay needed by people whose blood sugar drops quickly (bottom line), has an average drop (middle line), or comes down very slowly (top line). Remember, the blood sugar will drop quicker than usual because insulin for both the meal and for the high blood sugar are given.

The higher the blood sugar, the more High Blood Sugar Regular it takes to return the blood sugar to normal four to five hours later.

Doses of Regular for high blood sugars are correctly set when they bring high blood sugars back to normal in four to five hours.

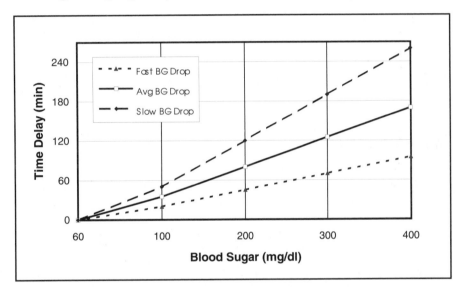

Figure 9.4 Delayed Eating With High Blood Sugars

WHAT HAPPENS WHEN THE INSULIN DOSE IS TOO LOW OR HIGH?

If not enough insulin is given, the blood sugar rises. Cells that need insulin don't get enough glucose. They lack fuel and the person feels tired. At the same time other cells which do not use insulin for the transport of glucose become exposed to high internal glucose levels which cause damage.

If too much insulin is given, the cells that use insulin will take in too much glucose. This drastically lowers the blood sugar, leaving the brain and nervous system with too little glucose to think clearly and maintain coordination.

Hope is the feeling you have that the feeling you have isn't permanent.

Jean Kerr

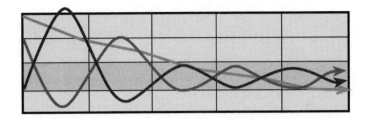

SPECIAL TIPS ON INSULIN DOSES AND ORAL AGENTS IN TYPE II DIABETES

10

Clean slates have their advantages and the same holds in treating diabetes. Replacement of insulin is more straightforward in Type I diabetes, where little insulin is being produced. In Type II, insulin usage is complicated by the person's own production and often by resistance to insulin. The internal production plus the unquantified resistance makes insulin doses harder to predict. One person may have mild resistance and need only a small dose to aid their internal production. Another person may require very large doses because they are very resistant to insulin. In this case, the second person may actually be producing more of their own insulin than the first!

Therapy is also complicated by a wide range of available medications to enhance the internal production of insulin, lower the internal production of glucose, or delay the rise of blood sugars following a meal.

In this chapter, we'll look at:

- How the "apple shape" creates insulin resistance
- Different stages of therapy in Type II diabetes
- The variety of oral agents that are available for treatment

WHEN APPLES AREN'T HEALTHY

Apples may be good for you, but an apple figure, with excess weight in the middle, isn't. The apple figure is quite common in people with Type IIr diabetes, and is occasionally seen in people with Type I diabetes. The risk for heart disease goes up two and a half times for men who have diabetes with the apple figure, but rises eightfold for women with this shape. Men and women with the apple figure are at the same high risk for heart disease, and over 70 percent will die from cardiovascular disease. One out of every four people in the United States has insulin resistance. Because of it, they are more prone to heart disease, even if they never actually develop diabetes.

Besides inherited genes, controllable lifestyle factors have been shown to create excess fat deposits in the middle. These include the use of alcohol (and yes, especially beer), smoking, stress, lack of exercise, eating fewer than three meals a day, and a diet high in fat or simple sugars.

Why Is the Apple Figure So Risky?

Fat cells in the abdomen release fat into the blood more easily than fat cells located elsewhere. Fat release from the abdomen begins three to four hours after the last meal compared to many more hours for fat cells in other areas of the body. This easy release shows up as higher triglyceride (TG) and free fatty acid levels. Free fatty acids themselves cause resistance to insulin.

Excess cardiac risks found when someone has an apple figure include: higher triglyceride levels, lower HDL (protective cholesterol), higher blood pressure, diabetes (usually Type IIr), and kidney disease. Often there is a family history of high blood pressure, heart disease, diabetes, or cholesterol problems.

Do You Have An Apple Figure?

To find out whether you have an apple figure, determine your waist-to-hip ratio. Measure around your waist with a tape measure an inch above the navel. Then measure your hips at their widest point. Divide your waist measurement by your hip measurement.

A ratio over 0.8 for women or over 1.0 for men suggests an unhealthy accumulation of fat in the middle. If you've got an apple figure, you can do the following to improve insulin sensitivity and to prevent health problems:

- Eat fewer calories and less fat
- Eat less, but more often
- Keep blood sugars normal
- Drink little or no alcohol
- Exercise regularly
- Don't smoke
- Reduce stress or manage it better

Skipping Meals

Is skipping meals healthy? Maybe not. When someone eats only once or twice a day, his body learns to store extra fat in an easy-to-access area (the abdomen) to get through those long periods with no eating. The fat stored in the middle is the quickly released variety. When you skip meals, and also during the overnight, more fat circulates in the blood with a greater risk for damage to blood vessels. Eating small amounts of carbohydrate through the day keeps fat release to a minimum and keeps the weight down because it lessens the need for fat storage in the abdomen.

HOW ORAL AGENTS AFFECT CONTROL AND INSULIN DOSES

There are three different types of oral agents now available that can be used to improve blood sugar control in Type II diabetes. The first type, called the sulfonylureas, includes several different drugs that have been available for over 35 years in the United States. The other two types were introduced into the United States in 1995. Each type works by different mechanisms, so different combinations can be tried to achieve excellent blood sugar control.

One advantage to having these choices is that treatments can be better tailored to meet the needs of a wide variety of individual blood sugar patterns. Another benefit is that with selective use of these medications, control can be achieved with lower doses of insulin and less risk for hypoglycemia.

The availability of the two new types, metformin and acarbose, which complement the blood sugar lowering effect of the sulfonylureas and of each other, has delayed or reduced the need for insulin in many people with Type II diabetes. Some individuals who have needed small doses of insulin have been able to come off it, or reduce their insulin doses, through judicious use of these three different classes of drugs.

Sulfonylureas

There are a number of sulfonylurea medications that have been in use for as long as 40 years. The older "first generation" medications include tolbutamide (Orinase), tolazamide (Tolinase), and chlorpropamide (Diabinese). These drugs work just as well as the newer ones in lowering the blood sugar, but because they bind to proteins in the blood, they are more prone to being dislodged which increases their activity, or to dislodging other medications that bind to the same proteins.

Diabinese, in particular, lasts longer in the blood and is more likely to cause a rare, but severe and long-lasting, type of hypoglycemia. Its use, particularly in older individuals, has greatly decreased because of this risk.

The newer "second generation" medications include glipizide (Glucotrol) and glyburide (Micronase, Glynase, and Diabeta). These are less likely to interact with other medications a person is using because they don't bind to proteins in the blood used by these other medications. This may be an advantage to individuals who are on other medications.

Micronase, Glynase, and Diabeta work best when taken twice a day, half before breakfast and half before dinner. If taken all at once, there is more chance for hypoglycemia. For some who have higher readings only at bedtime and breakfast, the medication may be required only before the evening meal. Glucotrol has a shorter action time than the others and may be less likely to cause hypoglycemia in those whose blood sugars are only mildly elevated.

These medications work best when taken at the same time each day. A person using oral agents should also be monitoring blood sugars to adjust doses properly. On average a single oral agent will work for five to seven years to control blood sugars.

The sulfonylureas work mainly by increasing insulin production from the beta cells in the pancreas. They also somewhat increase receptivity to insulin at the cell receptor level. They are effective for lowering the blood sugar. They also can cause low blood sugars, although this is less likely than with insulin injections.

Metformin

Metformin is a chemical cousin to the French lilac plant which was noted to lower blood sugars in the early 1900s. However, French lilac turned out to be too toxic for use in the treatment of diabetes. Metformin and its longer-acting relative, phenformin, were both developed in 1957. Unfortunately, phenformin reached the U.S. market first, and it caused several deaths. When this deadly side effect surfaced, phenformin was pulled from drugstore shelves worldwide. Metformin was tainted by a problem caused by its long-acting cousin. It was only cleared for use in Type II diabetes by the F.D.A. in 1995, but metformin has been widely used in Europe, Canada, and Mexico for many years.

Metformin, which has a much shorter action time, has a much lower risk for severe side effects. It appears to be quite safe to use by anyone who is otherwise healthy. It should not be used in those who abuse alcohol, who have congestive heart failure, or who have advanced kidney, liver, or lung disease. As noted, metformin has a long history of safe usage in other countries.

Metformin possesses some distinct advantages in treating diabetes. It works differently than the sulfonylureas, and the two classes of drugs work well together. Combined therapy leads to a greater fall in the blood sugars than either class by itself. Generally, the blood sugars fall about 20 percent farther when one class is added to the other.

Metformin works by reducing the production of glucose by the liver, enhancing the use of glucose by cells, and causing a mild slowdown in the absorption of glucose from food. The excess glucose produced by the liver is the major source for rising blood sugars in Type IIr diabetes, and is typically the reason for high blood sugars on waking in the morning. Metformin has several advantages:

- Lower blood sugars, especially after eating, without the risk of hypoglycemia

    Better lipids: total cholesterol and LDL levels drop about 10 percent, triglycerides drop by as much as 50 percent, and protective HDL levels rise about 10 percent[30, 31, 32]

- Plus a mild reduction in weight and blood pressure

One of the big advantages of metformin is that it reduces the amount of insulin needed to control the blood sugars in both Type I and Type II diabetes, although it has not been cleared for use in Type I diabetes.[33] For people with Type II diabetes already on insulin, this means that insulin doses must be reduced before metformin is started.

Acarbose

Like metformin, acarbose was released in the U.S. for use in Type II diabetes in 1995, It is produced under the brand name Precose and has been used in Europe for several years. Its action is quite different from sulfonylureas and metformin. By slowing the digestion of carbohydrates in the small intestine, the blood sugar rise after a meal is lessened. Acarbose works by inhibiting enzymes in the intestine that break carbohydrates down, so that glucose levels rise more slowly and the person's own internal production of insulin can more easily respond.

The way in which it works is also the major cause of its side effects. It generates what June Biermann and Barbara Toohey refer to as "social consequences": flatulence, abdominal distention, and diarrhea. These side effects can be minimized by a gradual increase in dosages over time. The side effects also tend to subside the longer the medication is used.

Like metformin, acarbose has advantages in that it does not cause low blood sugars or weight gain, nor does it raise insulin levels. Because it works in a different way, it can be added to the other two oral agents to improve blood sugar results.

WHY DO ORAL MEDICATIONS FAIL?

The oral agents that are used to treat Type II diabetes can greatly delay and in many cases eliminate completely the need for insulin. But they do not stop the progression of the underlying disease. If insulin resistance continues and the pancreas produces less and less of its own insulin over time, insulin injections become necessary to supply this critical hormone for health.

THE FUTURE PROMISE OF THIAZOLIDINEDIONES

This unpronounceable class of drugs holds great promise for the future in diabetes and perhaps in several other diseases. Resistance to insulin is an underlying cause of not only Type IIr diabetes, but also appears responsible for most cases of high blood pressure, and of the high triglycerides/low HDL cholesterol problem that puts many people at risk for heart disease.

Early drugs in this class, like Troglitazone, are being tested in Type II diabetes, and have been shown to lower blood sugar levels about 15 percent while *at the same time* lowering insulin levels by 20 percent. Blood pressure and triglyceride levels are also lowered, while HDL levels are raised.

These effects suggest that this class of drugs reverses insulin resistance, the key cause of Type II diabetes. These drugs might also be used to lower blood pressure and correct a cholesterol problem for which current medications are not terribly successful. Exactly how these drugs work is not yet clear, but the wide impact of this class of drugs on blood sugars, blood pressure, and cholesterol levels suggests we are closer to understanding the metabolic basis of insulin resistance. This should, in turn, improve medical interventions.

STAGES OF THERAPY

Several stages of therapy are used in Type II diabetes. These stages are briefly outlined.

Stage One: Diet And Exercise

When first diagnosed, some people with Type IIr diabetes are able to control their blood sugars by choosing healthier foods and participating in more exercise. Control is considered adequate when the fasting blood sugar stays below 130 mg/dl (7.2 mmol) and the HbA1c is no higher than one percentage point above the normal range of the lab. Weight loss is critical for success, but often a loss of about 10 pounds is all that is needed to bring the blood sugars into the normal range, especially when physical activity has been increased.

Some physicians may recommend using an oral agent at this stage even though the blood sugars are well-controlled. The thinking is that the beta cells are stressed from overproducing insulin, and that an oral agent may lessen this physical stress. Some research suggests this strategy may keep insulin production higher in later years, but more research is needed to truly answer this question.

Stage Two: Add An Oral Medication

Many people when first diagnosed with Type II diabetes are unable to control their blood sugars adequately even with the benefits of an improved diet, exercise, and some weight loss. Diabetes is usually diagnosed in adults only after the beta cells have already been stressed for 10, 20, or 30 years. True diabetes may already have been present for many years before the diagnosis is finally made. By the time the person finds out they have the disease, their insulin production may be too low to control the blood sugars. An oral medication is usually helpful at this point.

Oral medications should not be taken if the person is pregnant or considering pregnancy because of the chance for causing birth defects. A recent study found no increase in birth defects in women who were on a sulfonylurea prior to learning they were pregnant, but it is advisable to not run this unnecessary risk.

Stage Three: Add Another Oral Medication

Today, there are three separate medications to aid blood sugar control. Because they work in different ways, they can be used with one another to lower the blood sugars. So, before insulin is used, various combinations of the medications may be used to control blood sugars.

Stage Four: Add Insulin

When the maximum doses of one or more of the oral agents is being taken but the premeal blood sugars are over 130 mg/dl (7.2 mmol), or the HbA_{1c} is more than 1 to 1½ point or percent above the lab's upper limit for normal, insulin should be considered as the best way to control the blood sugars. Because the fasting blood sugar is often the highest one of the day, an evening dose of insulin is often the best option.

An injection before dinner of Regular combined with Lente or NPH is a great choice if both the bedtime and breakfast readings are high, as they often are in Type IIr diabetes. Another option is to first use NPH at bedtime to lower the fasting reading and see how well blood sugars through the rest of the day are controlled. This will often normalize the fasting blood sugar. An oral medication can then be used during the daytime hours to control the blood sugar. This last approach is often referred to as BIDS--Bedtime Insulin, Daytime Sulfonylureas. This therapy, which uses minimal insulin, sometimes helps in controlling weight.

If your blood sugars are high throughout the day, it is best to start with an injection of Regular and one of the long-acting insulins before breakfast and before dinner.

Currently, as many as 60 percent of those with Type II diabetes eventually go on to insulin. The body's resistance to insulin eventually becomes too much for the body to overcome. At this time, insulin may be added to oral agents or oral agents may be taken away and insulin used alone. As treatment options now available with Type II diabetes increase, we will expect to see a decrease in the number of people requiring insulin.

Someone did a study of the three most-often-heard phrases in New York City.
One is "Hey taxi."
Two is "What train do I take to get to Bloomingdales?"
And three is "Don't worry, it's only a flesh wound."

David Letterman

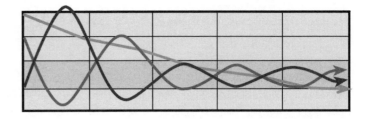

Tips On Insulin

11

This chapter provides information and practical tips for better use of insulin in controlling blood sugars. These tips make control easier, safer, and less expensive.

Injection Site Rotation

At one time, rotation of injection sites was recommended to prevent infections. But as insulin purity improved, infections vanished. Site rotation for this reason has become unnecessary. The abdomen has become the preferred injection site. It absorbs insulin rapidly and consistently from day to day, compared to muscle areas in the arms and legs. When insulin is injected into or near muscle sites, more variation in the blood sugar occurs, especially when these muscles are involved in exercise. The more consistent uptake of insulin from the abdomen improves blood sugar control.[34]

There are wide differences in how quickly insulin is picked up from different areas of the body. A general rule you can use on insulin timing: the lower in the trunk of the body you inject, the later in time that insulin will peak. One study found that the area above the navel was the fastest place to inject your insulin. Injected here, Regular insulin peaked in just over three hours in leaner people and at four hours in the overweight. Although relatively slow, this area was 30 to 60 minutes faster than the lower abdomen and 60 to 160 minutes faster than the thighs.[35]

These time differences can be used to your advantage. For meal coverage or to lower high blood sugars, the upper abdomen would be preferred. But for a safer lowering of a high bedtime reading, use of slower areas in the lower abdomen might be an advantage.

The absorption of insulin from the abdominal area is more consistent, especially when exercising.[36] But injection sites should always be rotated, even if only the abdomen is used. Injections can be placed at sites two fingerwidths away from the belly button extending to the sides, and from just below the rib cage to near the pubic area, basically anywhere you can "pinch an inch". Distributing sites in this way ensures that scarring will not interfere with insulin absorption. The hip area can also be used for backup, so to speak. But remember, for faster action use the higher regions.

Some people find an injection into the abdomen hard to think about, much less to do. But an injection into the abdomen is as easy and comfortable as any other area, if the mental block can be suppressed long enough to try it out. Some people benefit from the use of automatic injectors like Inject-Ease which keep the needle out of sight.

USE OF ALCOHOL AND REUSE OF SYRINGES

Cleansing the injection site with alcohol was recommended in the past as a way to prevent infections. However, alcohol is usually not required today because other advances have greatly reduced risks for infection: most insulins contain germicidal preservatives, and the small needles used today introduce very few bacteria through the skin.

Syringes are sometimes reused as a way to save money or protect the environment. Luckily, this appears to be quite safe, as infections have rarely been reported with this practice. Some helpful steps will ensure that an infection does not occur. Bacteria are transferred from two main sources: through the breath and by touch. Washing your hands with soap and water before starting reduces the bacterial counts and infection risk. Don't touch the syringe needle or the top of the insulin bottle. Keep the syringe and other equipment away from the nose and breath. These simple steps, together with the advances in needles and insulin, make an infection extremely unlikely.

Some people should never reuse syringes. Anyone with AIDS, leukemia or other diseases of the immune system, or anyone on immune suppressants like cyclosporin or prednisone, should use syringes only once. Also anyone who is careless about clean hands or sterile technique with needles and insulin bottles may be better off not reusing syringes.

> ### TIPS ON INSULIN
>
> - Insulin reactions and unexpected highs become less likely the more you test your blood sugars.
> - A varied lifestyle with set doses of insulin spells disaster. For greater freedom, give insulin frequently, with doses matched to your lifestyle.
> - Control is improved when insulin doses are smaller and given more often.
> - "Brittle" diabetes is created when insulin is given in the wrong amount or at the wrong time.
> - Regular insulin controls the first six hours after an injection; Lente or NPH controls the second six hours. Patterns of highs and lows can be corrected by understanding insulin timing.
> - Insulin doses are correctly set when blood sugars are stable and in the normal range.
> - Everyone needs to adjust their insulin doses occasionally
>
> **Know when to contact your physician!**

IS YOUR INSULIN OK?

Something everyone taking insulin should keep in mind is that insulin, a protein, can go bad when exposed to excess heat or freezing temperatures. Exposure to temperature extremes is more common when insulin is ordered from a central pharmacy located at a distance and shipped to your home. In transit, the insulin can be exposed to high or low temperatures causing degradation. This can happen even in transit to your local pharmacy. Someone who uses this insulin will become aware of the problem only when their blood sugars rise.

> ### HANDY DIABETES SUPPLIES
>
> **Insulin:**
> A short-acting insulin (Regular or Lispro), and a long-acting insulin (Lente, NPH, or Ultralente).
>
> **Lancets:**
> Ultrafine lancets and a lancing device
>
> **Blood sugar meter:**
> Meter and strips
>
> **Records:**
> Graphic charts or software for downloading data from your meter are recommended. See the last page for ordering information.
>
> **Low blood sugar treatment:**
> Glucagon injection kit, plus fast-acting carbs like glucose tablets, Sweet Tarts® or other dextrose candy, Monojel®

Luckily, insulin can be checked if you are unsure of its activity. A bottle of Regular can be grasped at the neck, turned upside down, and rocked gently back and forth. If the insulin is OK, it will be as clear as water with no clumps or particles in it and no clumps on the sides of the bottle. A bottle of long-acting insulin is first swirled gently to put it completely into solution. It can then be swirled. No clumps or particles should appear in the insulin or on the sides of the bottle. If there is any question, obtain a fresh bottle of insulin from your pharmacy with another lot number.

Diluting Insulin

Injections can be a problem for those who require only small doses (usually 25 or fewer units a day). People on small doses often have large variations in their blood sugars because they are so sensitive to insulin. This occasionally occurs in Type I and Type IIs diabetes. Luckily, insulin can be diluted with a diluent from the manufacturer. Dilution allows accurate delivery of smaller doses of insulin. Any inconvenience of dilution can be quickly offset by the improved blood sugar control and decreased risk for low blood sugars that result from more exact insulin delivery.[37]

Mixing Regular and Long-Acting Insulins

Research by Dr. John Galloway and others at Lilly suggests guidelines for mixing Regular with long-acting insulins.[38] It's best to take your injection right after mixing Regular and long-acting insulins. If the injection cannot be done right away, consider the following guidelines:

- If an injection is taken right away, Regular can be mixed with Lente or NPH with full retention of its normal activity.

- If delayed for 5 to 15 minutes after mixing, Regular retains better activity when mixed with Lente.

- If delayed for an hour or more, Regular retains better activity when mixed with NPH.

Premixed Insulins

Commercial combinations of Regular and NPH that have been premixed in a single bottle are available at many pharmacies. These mixtures combine 30 percent Regular and 70 percent NPH, or 50 percent Regular and 50 percent NPH. These premixed solutions are a real advantage for people who are visually impaired, or who are older and might have difficulty mixing insulins. The disadvantage is that these ratios cannot be altered once they are premixed. This does not allow someone on flexible insulin therapy to precisely alter their doses.

Can Different Long-Acting Insulins Be Combined?

Regular can be mixed with long-acting insulins, but what about mixing long-acting insulins with each other? Can different long- acting insulins be mixed in the same syringe or can they be taken at different times in the

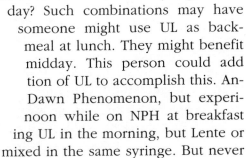

some advantages. For example, ground insulin but eat their largest from having more insulin available some Lente to their morning injec- other person who has a strong ences low blood sugars in the after- and bedtime, might benefit from us- NPH at bedtime. Lente and UL can be

day? Such combinations may have someone might use UL as back- meal at lunch. They might benefit midday. This person could add tion of UL to accomplish this. An- Dawn Phenomenon, but experi- noon while on NPH at breakfast ing UL in the morning, but Lente or mixed in the same syringe. But never

mix NPH directly with UL due to the different insulin binders they contain.

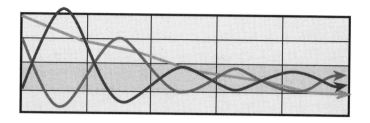

SEVERE HIGH BLOOD SUGARS AND KETOACIDOSIS

12

Severe high blood sugars and ketoacidosis are very serious medical problems seen in diabetes. These life-threatening conditions are most often seen in Type I or insulin-dependent diabetes where a person does not produce their own insulin. It is often present when a person first comes down with Type I diabetes.

High blood sugars and ketoacidosis can be triggered by bad insulin, forgetting to take insulin, a severe infection, or a severe illness. It may also occur in Type II diabetes under the stress of a severe illness like pneumonia or a heart attack. In children and adolescents with Type I diabetes, they can sometimes be triggered by growth spurts that make the body need more insulin. When an infection or severe illness is causing the problem, the high blood sugars will be difficult to bring down until the underlying problem is dealt with.

High blood sugars can exist for some time without triggering ketoacidosis. Ketoacidosis starts whenever insulin levels in the body go very low. When insulin is low, glucose, the body's first choice for energy, cannot be used as fuel. Instead, the body starts burning fat even though glucose is quite high in the blood.

Burning fat might sound like a good thing, especially if you are trying to lose weight. But this excessive use of fat turns out to be quite unhealthy because high levels of ketones and acidity are created in the blood. Although ketones are a normal byproduct of fat metabolism, when they are at high levels they cause the blood to become highly acidic which leads to nausea and vomiting. The vomiting plus the accompanying high blood sugars leads to dehydration. When acidity and dehydration are combined, it is quite serious and may cause death.

SYMPTOMS

Early symptoms of ketoacidosis include tiredness, great thirst, frequent urination, dry skin, a fruity odor to the breath, abdominal pain, and nausea. Late symptoms include vomiting, shortness of breath and rapid breathing as the body tries to clear the bloodstream of ketones and high blood sugars. These symptoms are due to the ketone poisoning and should never be ignored. As soon as a person begins to vomit or has difficulty breathing, immediate treatment in an emergency room is required to prevent coma and possible death.

Everyone with diabetes needs to know how to recognize and treat ketoacidosis. Ketones travel from the blood into the urine and can be detected in the urine with ketone test strips available at any pharmacy. Ketone strips should always be kept on hand, but stored in a dry area and replaced as soon as they become outdated.

Check the urine for ketones whenever a blood sugar reading is 300 mg/dl or higher, if a fruity odor is detected in the breath, if abdominal pain is present, if nausea or vomiting is occurring, or if you are breathing rapidly and short of breath. If a moderate or large amount of ketones are detected on the test strip, ketoacidosis is present and immediate treatment is required.

TREATMENT

To treat ketoacidosis, you must drink lots of fluid to prevent dehydration, and take extra amounts of Regular insulin to bring the blood sugars down. The dehydration is caused by excess urination due to high blood sugars and can be quickly worsened if vomiting starts due to excess ketones. If possible, start with a large quantity of water or other noncaloric or low caloric fluid, and then continue to drink at least 8 ounces every 30 minutes until the blood sugar is again normal. Sports drinks like Gatorade or water with a pinch of potassium-based Nu-Salt are helpful for replacing potassium in ketoacidosis.

If nausea or vomiting keep you from drinking fluids, call your physician and immediately go to an emergency room for treatment. Ask your physician the action you should take with each ketone strip reading.

To lower high blood sugars, give extra injections of Regular insulin. It

---

How To Treat Ketoacidosis

- Check urine for ketones whenever blood sugars go over 300 mg/dl (16.7 mmol).

- Drink a large amount of non-caloric or low caloric fluids immediately, followed by 8 to 12 oz. every 30 minutes. Gatorade and similar fluids are good because they help restore potassium levels.

- Take extra Regular insulin every 3 hours until blood sugars are below 200 mg/dl (11 mmol).

- If nausea starts, call your physician.

- *If vomiting starts or you are unable to drink fluids, call your physician and go to an emergency room immediately.*

---

helps to know how far your blood sugar drops on each unit of Regular insulin so you know how much extra insulin to give. Doses for High Blood Sugar Regular can be found in Chapter 16. If you want to lower the blood sugar faster, you can inject Regular into the upper abdomen or into the intramuscular areas of the inner biceps or thigh. Discuss this with your physician.

If the urine test shows that moderate or large amounts of ketones are present, much larger doses of insulin than usual may be needed, often one and a half to two times the usual doses. Check your blood sugar hourly until control has been regained. Be sure to check with your physician for the doses of Regular insulin to take and how often to take them.

Any occurrence of ketoacidosis should raise a red flag. Unless there is a clear reason for the ketoacidosis, such as an illness or an infection, a serious problem exists. Insulin doses may be too low or you may need to know more about how to use insulin for blood sugar control. Discuss any problems you have regarding high blood sugars or ketoacidosis with your physician so problems can be quickly resolved and prevented from happening again.

**Taking insulin to bring down a high blood sugar is important,
but staying hydrated is often MORE important!**

SETTING YOUR INSULIN DOSES

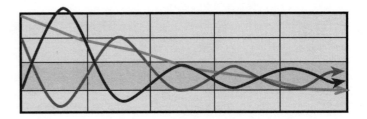

STARTING DOSES

13

The first thing to determine before starting flexible insulin therapy is how much insulin is needed each day. This is also called the total daily insulin dose or the "Big I" as Lois Jovanovic-Peterson, M.D., calls it. This total daily need for insulin can only be estimated at first.

In this chapter, we'll show:

- How to estimate your total daily need for insulin
- How to estimate starting doses for long-acting and Regular insulins.

Your physician/health care team will help you make these estimates using two different guides. Formulas exist to estimate your total insulin need. These formulas give a close approximation of the total daily insulin dose with Type I diabetes, but are not as accurate in Type II diabetes. Formulas don't reveal how much of this dose you'll need in your long-acting versus Regular insulins, nor how to split the long-acting insulin into morning and evening doses. Your physician and health care team have to be involved to make the precise adjustments needed and to instruct you in how to make these determinations for yourself.

STANDARD FORMULAS BASED ON BODY WEIGHT

To make a rough estimate based on your weight, use the first column in Table 13.1 to find your weight. Then look in that row at Columns 4, 5 and 6 to find one estimates for:

1. Your initial long-acting insulin dose
2. The ratio of Regular to grams of carbohydrate in meals
3. The number of points your blood sugar is likely to drop on each unit of Regular.

STANDARD FORMULAS BASED ON YOUR PREVIOUS INSULIN DOSES

Another way to estimate these insulin needs is from the amount of insulin you've actually been using each day. This method is most accurate if your control has been fairly good on these doses. You need only add up the amount of insulin you've been using in the past. Add up the total insulin you use each day in your injections, including doses of both Regular and Lente, NPH or Ultralente. Look in column 3 of Table 13.1 for the row that has this total insulin dose. Then look across at columns 4, 5 and 6 to find your estimated starting doses for long-acting and Regular insulins based on your previous insulin doses.

If your blood sugar has been well-controlled on injections in the past, the total dose of insulin you've been using will be very close to the total dose you'll need with flexible therapy.

Setting Your Insulin Doses

But if your control has not been great, your physician/health care team's experience can give you a better estimate for these starting doses.

These starting doses are then tested and readjusted to match your actual need. Periodic retesting is also needed because daily life never remains the same, and along with changes in daily life come changes in glucose control and insulin need.

At times these estimates don't agree. If these estimated doses do not agree, it is almost always best to start with the lower number. One exception to using the lower dose may occur if the blood sugars in the past have been well-controlled, but on a dose of insulin that's greater than that recommended by your weight. If you are faced by this situation, discuss it with your physician before attempting any change.

Factors such as food choices, activity, general health, age, sensitivity to insulin, and production of hormones can affect the need for insulin. If your weight is above your ideal weight,

Estimates For Starting Insulin Doses On Flexible Insulin Therapy					
1	2	3	4	5	6
Row	Your Weight (lbs)	Your Previous Total Daily Insulin Dose On 1 or 2 Injections	Long-Acting Insulin L/NPH/UL: (units/day)	Carb Regular: 1 unit of Reg. for each:	High Blood Sugar Regular: 1 unit of Reg. for each:
1	80	18 units	8 to 11	24 grams	90 pts > target
2	90	21 units	9 to 12	21 grams	80 pts > target
3	100	23 units	10 to 14	18 grams	70 pts > target
4	110	26 units	12 to 16	17 grams	60 pts > target
5	120	30 units	13 to 18	15 grams	50 pts > target
6	130	32 units	13 to 19	15 grams	47 pts > target
7	140	35 units	16 to 21	13 grams	43 pts > target
8	150	37 units	17 to 22	12 grams	40 pts > target
9	160	40 units	18 to 24	11 grams	37 pts > target
10	180	45 units	20 to 27	10 grams	33 pts > target
11	200	54 units	24 to 32	8 grams	28 pts > target
12	220	60 units	27 to 36	7 grams	25 pts > target
13	240	66 units	30 to 40	6 grams	23 pts > target

Table 13.1 Estimated Doses for Long-acting and Regular Insulins based on Weight and Previous Total Daily Insulin Doses (Type I Diabetes)

Starting doses must always be discussed with your physician before testing begins.

if you eat a diet with a higher fat content, if you exercise only at your desk, if you have been in poor control for some time, or if you produce extra stress hormones that block insulin, you will need more insulin. If you're a teenager with high hormone levels aiding your growth, you may need much more insulin. Your physician/health care team's familiarity with these factors allows them to help you make accurate estimates of your own insulin requirements.

Using Table 13.1, fill in Table 13.2 on this page to determine your estimated starting doses for long-acting insulin, Carb Regular, and High Blood Sugar Regular. If you're already on multiple injections, use this information to evaluate your current insulin doses. Be sure to discuss these estimated doses with your physician/health care team before changing anything. Be aware also that these

---

Worksheet To Determine Starting Insulin Dose

1. What is your weight? _____ lbs.

2. In column #2 find the row that is nearest to your weight: Row # _____

3. How much total insulin do you use each day? I average: _____ units/day

4. In column #3 find the row that is nearest to your total insulin dose: Row # _____

5. Which row number is lower? Row # _____

6. Using the values from this row, my starting insulin doses will be:

   a. My long-acting insulin doses is between:

      _____ units and _____ units a day.

   b. My Carb Regular is 1 Regular for each:

      _____ grams of carbohydrate.

   c. My High Blood Sugar Regular is:

      One unit of Regular for each _____ points above my target blood sugar.

Table 13.2 See Table 13.1 to fill in this Worksheet

---

starting insulin doses might need to be reduced soon after you start them, especially if your blood sugar control has been poor in the past and improves quickly. Better blood sugars often lead to a decrease in the need for insulin.[7, 39]

More long-acting insulin in the evening insulin dose may be suggested for the initial test by your physician/health care team if you have a Dawn Phenomenon. Most people with diabetes have either a Dawn Phenomenon if they're Type I, or a high morning reading due to the insulin resistance of Type IIr diabetes. The Dawn Phenomenon is frequently found in Type I diabetes due to a normal nighttime release of growth hormone. High blood sugars at breakfast are often seen in Type IIr diabetes because of insulin resistance and the release of fatty acids from the abdomen during the night. People who have their highest readings at breakfast will need to adjust the timing and the amount of the evening dose of long-acting insulin to accommodate this need. On average, an increase of 20 percent in the early morning insulin dose is needed to offset a Dawn Phenomenon.[40]

In a small group of people who have a very strong Dawn Phenomenon, even multiple injections will not work to control the morning blood sugar. If you fall into this group, you may want to discuss using an insulin pump with your physician. The precise delivery of Regular insulin from a pump is superior to injections in controlling an early morning rise in blood sugar levels, and this effect is seen both on waking blood sugars[41] and into the early afternoon hours.[42]

SENSITIVITY TO INSULIN

To set your insulin doses correctly, it helps to know how sensitive to insulin you are. For those with Type I diabetes, insulin sensitivity can be estimated by filling in the blanks below:

1. Your weight in pounds divided by 4   =   _____ units

2. Your total daily insulin dose (all insulins)   =   _____ units

The answer from line 1 is your estimated need for insulin. If your actual insulin dose on line 2 is close to this number, and you have good control, you have a normal sensitivity to insulin. If line 2 is less than line 1 (and your control is good), you have excellent insulin sensitivity.

If line 2 is much greater than line 1, your insulin sensitivity may be less than average or you may be on too much insulin. (Are you having frequent insulin reactions?) If insulin sensitivity is low, the tips in Chapter 2 for the apple figure can help to improve it.

With *Type II diabetes*, determining sensitivity to insulin is more complicated because individuals vary in the amount of insulin they produce themselves and in their degree of insulin resistance. Insulin sensitivity helps to determine the total daily insulin dose, including the background insulin, Carbohydrate Regular, and High Blood Sugar Regular.

ONE EXAMPLE OF USING THE WORKSHEET

Frances has Type I diabetes, weighs 160 pounds and is close to her ideal body weight. Her current control on two shots a day has been erratic, with frequent insulin reactions. She has been taking 10 Regular and 32 NPH before breakfast, and 10 Regular and 8 NPH before dinner, for a total daily insulin dose of 60 units.

Using her total dose (Column 3 in Table 13.1), she finds the estimate for her starting insulin doses in Row 12. From Column 2 she finds the estimate for her starting insulin doses based on a weight of 160 pounds in Row 9.

The sample worksheet (Table 13.3) shows how Frances determined her insulin doses. Note that she chose to start on the lower doses suggested in Row 9. This Row has lower starting doses and would be preferred because of her frequent lows on 60 units of insulin a day. This represents a considerable reduction in her insulin doses. However, when lows occur, they won't be as frequent or as severe. The insulin doses can of course be raised if testing shows these lower doses are not adequate.

Worksheet To Determine Starting Insulin Doses

1. What is your weight?   <u>160</u> lbs.

2. In column #2 find the row that is nearest to your weight: Row # <u>9</u>

3. How much total insulin do you use each day? I average: <u>60</u> units/day

4. In column #3 find the row that is nearest to your total insulin dose: Row # <u>12</u>

5. Which row number is lower?   Row # <u>9</u>

6. Using the values from this row, my starting insulin doses will be:

   a. My long-acting insulin doses is between:

      <u>18</u> units and <u>24</u> units a day.

   b. My Carb Regular is 1 Regular for each:

      <u>11</u> grams of carbohydrate.

   c. My High Blood Sugar Regular is:

   One unit of Regular for each <u>37</u> points above my target blood sugar.

Table 13.3 One Example Using the Worksheet

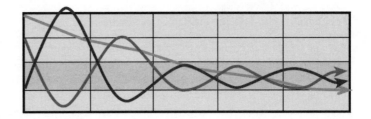

FINDING THE RIGHT LONG-ACTING INSULIN DOSE

14

In Chapter 13 you learned how to find your correct total insulin dosage. This chapter will show you how to find the best long-acting insulin doses for you and how to use them to:

- Keep the blood sugars constant
- Match the Dawn Phenomenon
- Prevent unnecessary highs and lows

Whenever a change is made in the long-acting insulin doses, testing of the new dose cannot be done right away, but has to be delayed until the changes from the new dosage is seen in insulin levels in the bloodstream. This typically takes 30 to 48 hours following a change in doses of Lente or NPH insulins, and 60 to 72 hours following a change in the doses of Ultralente.

WHICH LONG-ACTING INSULIN IS BEST?

Which long-acting insulin is best for you? Each insulin has different features:

NPH has a faster peak than Lente. Ideal for use at bedtime to match a Dawn Phenomenon.

Lente has a later and more rounded peak than NPH. May have advantages in providing "flatter" background insulin levels, and for possible use before dinner to cover the Dawn Phenomenon.

UL has a "flatter" peak than NPH or Lente. Ideal for those who have little or no Dawn Phenomenon.

WHEN SHOULD THE EVENING LONG-ACTING INSULIN BE GIVEN?

Should the evening long-acting insulin be given before dinner or at bedtime? The decision on the long-acting insulin to use and the time in the evening to give it depends on whether you have nighttime insulin reactions and on whether you have high blood sugars in the morning. The questions below help determine the type and timing of the long-acting insulin.

Nighttime Lows?	Morning Highs?	Best Choice
no	no	UL or L before dinner or at bedtime
yes	no	L or NPH at bedtime, or UL before dinner
no	yes	NPH at bedtime or L before dinner
yes	yes	NPH or L at bedtime

TESTING THE LONG-ACTING INSULIN

Always consult with your physician/health care team to select your starting morning and evening long-acting insulin doses. Once a starting dose and type of long-acting insulin has been selected, it is tested for accuracy. The goal here is to find both morning and evening doses of long-acting insulin that will keep the blood sugar relatively stable, or let it fall only slightly when no food is eaten. The testing is split into three times during the day for convenience.

The suggested times for night and day background insulin tests match typical working and sleeping hours. Those who work odd hours, a nightshift or varied shifts will need to adjust the timing of the tests to their own sleep and work schedules.

The overnight tests are done before the daytime tests because other activities that affect blood sugars, like exercise and eating, are suspended during the night, and because control of the waking blood sugar is the most important thing you can do for your overall control. Tests are repeated until desirable results are obtained on two or more occasions with the same dose of evening long-acting insulin.

What advantage is there to correctly setting the nighttime insulin? The obvious one is avoiding an insulin reaction in the middle of the night or waking up thirsty and tired from a high blood sugar. Also a steady blood sugar in a desirable range through the night is the first step to having normal readings through the day. You experience a full night of sound sleep and your daytime control is easier when you wake up with a normal reading.

Testing of the daytime long-acting insulin doses is split into two segments. The first half of the daytime test is done between waking and mid-afternoon. The second test is done on another day from mid-afternoon to bedtime. Each test is repeated until desirable results are obtained on two or more occasions with the same dose. Starting background insulin doses are adjusted as needed until they keep the blood sugar stable through the entire day.

With the Correct Nighttime Long-Acting Insulin, You Can:

• Go to bed with a normal blood sugar, eat little or no bedtime snack, and wake up with a normal blood sugar in the morning. (Assuming your dinner Regular is no longer active and you've had no excess activity that day.)

• Correct any high bedtime blood sugars and be confident that you will wake up with a good reading in the morning.

• Rest peacefully. You, your spouse, your parents, children, friends, room-mates, and physician/health care team will all sleep better knowing you're unlikely to have an insulin reaction during the night.

If doses of the daytime long-acting insulin change significantly due to this testing, testing and readjustment of the nighttime dose may have to be repeated. Wait a few days between tests to see what affect your new setting has on your blood sugars.

During testing, always keep in mind the time at which you expect your long-acting insulin to peak in activity (refer to Chapter 9). Test the blood sugar more often during this peak time to avoid a low blood sugar. Remember: finding the right long-acting insulin dose is the most important step in controlling your blood sugars.

PREPARATION

Testing the nighttime long-acting insulin dose takes some preparation. Don't try this test after you've had a severe insulin reaction, major emotional stress or unusually strenuous exercise during the day. Both major insulin reactions and emotional stress release stress hormones into the blood that continue to raise the blood sugar level for several hours afterward. Strenuous exercise has just the opposite effect by enhancing insulin's action over the next several hours. Events like these can distort your results if they happen on the day the nighttime dose is tested.

THE NIGHTTIME LONG-ACTING INSULIN

Follow the directions in Table 14.1 to prepare for the nighttime insulin test. Suggested times for blood sugar tests can be tailored to your own work and sleep hours. The dinner or bedtime long-acting insulin is then adjusted from these blood sugar results. Raise or lower the dose as instructed until you find a dose that keeps your blood sugar relatively steady on at least two consecutive tests.

Be certain to check your starting doses with your physician/health care team before the test, especially if you have any doubts about your doses, about how to interpret the readings, or whether to change the timing or amount of your insulin. Don't forget the 2 a.m. test! This middle-of-the-night blood sugar is critical for determining whether the nighttime long-acting insulin needs to be increased or decreased, and when is the best time to give the injection. Once you have obtained desirable results on at least two occasions with the same dose, stay at that dose for a few days and then test the daytime long-acting insulin dose.

Note that the blood sugar at the start of the test must be between 100 and 150 mg/dl (5.6 to 8.3 mmol). Although the upper part of this testing range is above that generally recommended, it allows room for the blood sugar to fall if the insulin dose has been set too high. Once the long-acting insulin has been correctly set, ideal blood sugars can be more safely achieved and maintained. The correct nighttime insulin keeps the blood sugar from rising, and lowers the blood sugar no more than 30 points overnight.

THE DAYTIME LONG-ACTING INSULIN

Table 14.1 also gives directions for testing the daytime long-acting insulin. For these tests you'll want to start either when you get up in the morning, or when at least five hours have passed since your last dose of Regular, and three hours after your last food was eaten. This ensures that only the background insulin will be affecting the blood sugars.

Testing the daytime insulin is done in two parts for convenience and accuracy. Fasting is required, and it's easier to fast a half day rather than a whole day.

Having the daytime long-acting insulin correctly set allows you to:

- Skip meals when necessary
- Eat meals late with less worry about an insulin reaction
- Give doses of Regular that will precisely cover carbohydrates and high blood sugars

People often have reservations about skipping meals for these tests. Some find it difficult to imagine going a few hours without food. But the human body is amazingly adaptive and will survive this ordeal. Some object: "They've always told me to eat when I take any insulin." The beauty of flexible therapy is that this is no longer necessary (except perhaps for an occasional snack).

Remember, a correctly set dose for the long-acting insulin is the most important step in having normal blood sugars. A few hours of fasting is a small price to pay for this success. If you are concerned about having a reaction on your current doses of long-acting insulin, check your blood sugar more often and consult with your physician/health care team about starting your test on a lower dose.

Note again your blood sugar at the start of the test should be between 100 and 150 mg/dl (5.6 to 8.3 mmol) in case the insulin dose is set too high and the blood sugar falls. Once the long-acting insulin has been correctly set, ideal blood sugars can be more safely achieved and maintained.

First Half Of The Daytime Test

The first half of the daytime test starts when you wake in the morning and ends in the mid-afternoon. Basically, eat no breakfast and a late lunch, unless a low blood sugar occurs. There must be nothing interfering with your blood sugars, like a recent meal or a dose of Regular insulin.

Do this test on a day when you'll be at your normal level of activity, so that extra work or exercise won't themselves be lowering the blood sugar. Similar to the nighttime test, there must be no strenuous exercise, excess stress, or a major insulin reaction in the hours preceding the test. Repeat the test until you have had the same desirable results on at least two occasions with the same dose of long-acting insulin.

Second Half of the Daytime Test

The second half of the test is done on a different day, a few days after the first. It covers the late afternoon and evening. For the second half, have an early lunch and start the test five hours after you take the Carb Regular for lunch. Then eat dinner close to bedtime and take your Carb Regular to cover it, although a smaller dose than usual will help to avoid a nighttime reaction.

Testing at this time checks primarily the morning dose of long-acting insulin. Consult with your physician/health care team regarding the starting dose for the long-acting insulin. Test and adjust this dose until you have the same desirable results on two consecutive tests.

Precautions

- Test your blood sugar often, especially if you think it may drop.

- If your blood sugar drops below 70 mg/dl (3.9 mmol), eat at least 15 grams of carbohydrate and end the test. Discuss lowering your dose with your physician/health care team. If the blood sugar drop is rapid, a large decrease in the long-acting insulin dose is needed. If the drop occurs slowly, a small decrease is needed.

- If your blood sugar goes over 200 mg/dl (11.1 mmol), take High Blood Sugar Regular to correct the high blood sugar and end the test. Discuss raising your insulin dose with your physician/health care team. If this blood sugar rise is rapid, a large increase in the long-acting insulin is needed. If the rise occurs slowly, a small increase is needed.

With experience, you can make changes whenever needed. Consult with your physician/health care team any time you're uncertain what your test results mean.

Steps For Testing The Long-Acting Insulin			
Test	Preparation	Test The Blood Sugar	What If The Blood Sugar Rises Or Falls?
Overnight Test	Take dinner Regular at least 5 hours before bed. Sugar between 100 and 150 (5.6 to 8.3 mmol) at bedtime to start.	at bedtime, at 2 AM, and on waking	If the sugar rises over 30 points (1.7 mmol) during this period, raise long-acting insulin by 1 or 2 units. If the sugar falls more than 30 points, lower long-acting insulin by 1 or 2 units. Retest.
First Daytime Test---no breakfast and a late lunch	On waking in the AM, start the test. Sugar between 100 and 150 (5.6 to 8.3 mmol) to start.	every 1 to 2 hours	Same
Second Daytime Test---early lunch and a late dinner	No Regular for 5 hours and no eating for 3 hrs before start of test. Sugar between 100 and 150 (5.6 to 8.3 mmol) to start.	every 1 to 2 hours	Same

Table 14.1 How to set doses for the long-acting insulin

TIPS ON THE LONG-ACTING INSULIN DOSE:

- Set and test the long-acting insulin doses before testing the Regular insulin doses. The background insulin requirement has to be correctly matched before doses of Regular can be correctly set for carbohydrate or high blood sugars.

- The best dose for the long-acting insulin is one that causes the blood sugar to stay stable or to drop slightly over several hours while not eating. Those who experience a slight drop in their blood sugar overnight should eat a bedtime snack. (Do *not* take Carb Regular for this.) Carbohydrate will be needed when the bedtime blood sugar is less than 80 mg/dl to 100 mg/dl (5.0 to 5.6 mmol), or when extra exercise has occurred that day.

- Signs that the long-acting insulin dose is too high:

    Frequent lows or a pattern of lows when the long-acting insulin is peaking

    Blood sugar drops when a meal is skipped

- Signs that the long-acting insulin dose is too low:

    Frequent highs

    Blood sugar rises when a meal is skipped

- Quick check of the long-acting insulin: Does the daily total for all the long-acting insulin doses make up about half (45 to 60 percent) of the total daily insulin dose?

- Coverage for carbohydrates and correction of high readings are made by changing Regular rather than the long-acting insulin used for background coverage.

Humility is no substitute for a good personality.

Jon Winokur

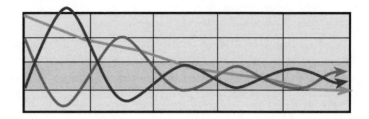

SETTING THE CARB REGULAR

15

Regular insulin normally makes up 40 to 55 percent of the total daily insulin dose. It is used to balance the carbohydrate in meals and snacks. When done properly, this balancing of food with injections of Regular before each meal allows great freedom in food choices and in meal timing. An individual's ratio of Regular to carbohydrate is determined by their sensitivity to insulin which, in turn, is affected largely by body weight and physical activity.

More weight and less physical activity translate into a lower sensitivity to insulin. About 25 percent of the U.S. population, including 70 percent of adults who have Type IIr diabetes and most people who have an apple-shaped figure, have some degree of insulin resistance. Additional clues to insulin resistance, besides diabetes, include a high triglyceride level on the cholesterol test, high blood pressure, an elevated uric acid level, or a close relative with Type II diabetes. If insulin resistance is present, more insulin is needed to control blood sugars and to cover carbohydrates. Occasionally an individual who is overweight and severely insulin-resistant may require as much as one unit of Regular for every two to five grams of carbohydrate.

Not everyone who gets diabetes as an adult is resistant to insulin, of course. Many people with Type IIs are thin and quite sensitive to insulin. These individuals may need only one unit of Regular for every 20 grams of carbohydrate. On average, most people with Type I diabetes require a unit of Regular for every 8 to 16 grams of carbohydrate. If you have not done so already, you can use Table 13.1 in Chapter 13 to estimate your own starting ratio of Regular to grams of carbohydrate.

The ratio of Regular to carbohydrate may vary slightly for different meals of the day. A unit of Regular often covers less carbohydrate (fewer

> **Reminder**
>
> Always set and test your long-acting insulin before attempting to determine your Carb Regular. How much Regular is needed for meals and high blood sugars can only be determined *after the background or long-acting insulin has been correctly set.*

grams) at breakfast compared to other meals. This decreased insulin sensitivity in the morning results from the production of more glucose-raising hormones, especially growth hormone, in the early morning hours. Doses of Regular that are given early in the day for breakfast and lunch begin to overlap during the afternoon and evening hours due to their six to seven hour action time.[43] Because of its faster activity and shorter action time, the new Lispro insulin speeds the entry of insulin into the blood to counteract glucose-raising hormones and also avoids much of the problem caused by overlapping doses of insulin.

SETTING THE REGULAR TO CARB RATIO

Similar to the background insulin dose determination, the first estimate for Regular to carbohydrate ratio is based on weight or on the previous average 24-hour insulin doses (whichever gives the lower estimate). This ratio of Regular to carbohydrate can then be adjusted as needed for extra activity, for foods with a low glycemic index, and so on.

To determine how much Regular to give for a meal, count the grams of carbohydrate in the meal you plan to eat. Carb counting is a simple way to optimize blood sugar control and is explained in Chapter 8 and Appendix A.

TIMING THE CARB REGULAR

Although the correct ratio of a unit of Regular to grams of carbohydrate is critical to good blood sugar control, another important factor is the timing of the dose: how long before a meal or large snack the injection is given. When a person neglects taking her Regular soon enough before eating, the blood sugar can spike to very high levels at one or two hours afterwards. Regular insulin works best when it is given 30 to 45 minutes before eating, or even earlier if the blood sugar is high. And as noted, when Lispro becomes available, it should help avoid this common problem.

There are times when Regular cannot be given at the appropriate time before eating. If you plan to eat out at a restaurant or the timing of a meal is uncertain, you may not be able to give the full dose of Carb Regular 30 to 45 minutes before eating. But you might consider a partial injection, perhaps half of the total amount that's anticipated for the meal. Then give the remaining Regular when eating actually begins and the carbohydrate count is more certain.

This partial dose allows the blood insulin level to begin rising by the time eating starts, but reduces the risk of a low blood sugar. The same technique can be used if the timing of a meal is known but the amount of carbohydrate is not. Fast-acting carbohydrates should always be available in case the blood sugar drops before the meal is actually served.

TESTING CARBOHYDRATE COVERAGE

The Regular to Carbohydrate Test begins with an estimate of the ratio of Regular to grams of carbohydrate. A beginning estimate can be found in Table 13.1 but this should always be checked with a personal recommendation from your physician/health care team. The flow chart on the next page shows how to test this ratio to see if it is correct for you. From these tests, the starting ratio is adjusted as needed until you find your own correct ratio.

The correct ratio of Regular to grams of carbohydrate will return the blood sugar to within 30 points (1.7 mmol) of the original blood sugar five hours after eating. Blood sugars are tested at two, three, and four hours after eating to reduce the risk of hypoglycemia. Repeat the test several times to determine the most accurate ratio for you.

Remember that slight variations in your ratio may occur for food eaten at different times during the day. Also, foods that have the same amount of carbohydrate but different glycemic indexes may require different doses of Regular. For instance, 50 grams of carbohydrate from kidney beans is unlikely to require as much Regular insulin as 50 grams eaten as pizza.

If you have a low blood sugar just two to three hours after your injection, your ratio of Regular to carbs is likely to be much too high. Too much Regular for not enough carbohydrate causes a rapid drop in the blood sugar. This requires a larger change in the Regular to Carbohydrate Ratio than if the low occurred four or five hours after eating. For instance, if you were using 1 Regular for each 12 grams, add two or three grams to the carbohydrate, so you're now using 1 Regular for each 14 or 15 grams. This gives you less Regular for the same amount of carbohydrate and makes a low blood sugar less likely.

If the low blood sugar happens four to five hours after the injection, the ratio of Regular to carbohydrate is close and only needs slight adjustment. Add 1 to the carbohydrate number, so that instead of 1 Regular for each 12 grams, it now becomes 1 Regular for each 13 grams.

Once you've found a ratio that normally works best for you, but you have a high or low blood sugar after a particular meal or snack, consider:

- Did you count the carbs carefully in the meal?
- Did you take your shot at least 30 minutes before eating?

Note that some change in this ratio may be needed for different meals during the day. A unit of Regular often covers less carbohydrate at breakfast than at other meals. An example would be one unit of Regular for every eight grams of carbohydrate at breakfast rather than one Regular for every 10 grams for the rest of the day. During pregnancy, more insulin is often needed for the same amount of carbohydrate due to changes that occur in carrying a child.

TIPS ON CARB REGULAR

- Test the Regular to Carbohydrate Ratio only after the long-acting insulin doses have been tested and accurately set.
- The correct ratio of Regular to grams of carbohydrate returns the blood sugar to within 30 points of the original blood sugar five hours after eating.
- The dose of Carb Regular is determined before each meal or snack by the carbohydrate contained in that meal, after consideration is given to the current blood sugar and any planned activities.
- Normal doses of Regular need to change when ketoacidosis, an infection, a change in weight, or a change in physical activity occur. Test more often when giving doses of Regular in these circumstances.
- Signs of an incorrect ratio for the Carb Regular:
  —Too little Regular: the blood sugar is OK before meals or snacks, but frequently goes high after meals and stays high before the next meal (or at bedtime).
  —Too much Regular: the blood sugar is OK before meals or snacks, but low blood sugars frequently happen two to four hours after food is eaten.
- Quick check of the Carb Regular: Do doses of Regular during the day make up 40 to 55 percent of the total daily insulin dose?

How to Test Your Regular to Carbohydrate Ratio

Preparation

1. With Table 13.1 and your doctor's advice, decide how many **grams of carbohydrate** will by covered by **one unit of Regular**.

2. Remember: your long-acting insulin must already have been tested.

3. Take no Regular for five hours and no food for three hours before testing starts.

✔ Check your **starting blood sugar** 30 minutes before eating. 80 to 120 mg/dl is ideal. 70 to 150 is OK.

Decide how many carbs you will eat.
Then determine how much Regular is needed to cover these carbs.
(Divide the grams of carbs you plan to eat
by the carb number from number 1 above.)

At mealtime, eat your meal as planned

✔ Check your blood sugar at two and three hours.
Has it risen 40 to 80 points (2.2 to 4.4 mmol)?

NO   **YES** ▼   **NO**

Less than 40 point (2.2 mmol) rise?	✔ Check at four hours to make sure the blood sugar is not low.	**More than 80 pt. (4.4 mmol) rise?**
End the test and eat if below 70 mg/dl (4.4 mmol). If above 80 mg/dl, test more often to avoid a low.		End the test and correct blood sugar if above 240 (15 mmol). If below 240, continue.

✔ Check at five hours:

Over 30 points below starting blood sugar?	**Within 30 points (1.7 mmol) of starting blood sugar?**	**Over 30 points above starting blood sugar?**
Retest using a higher carb number (i.e., if it was 1R/12 grams, retest with 1R/13 grams.	**You have the correct ratio.**	Retest using a lower carb number (i.e., if it was 1R/12 grams, retest with 1R/11 grams.

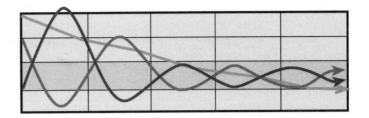

SETTING THE HIGH BLOOD SUGAR REGULAR

16

Besides covering carbohydrate, Regular insulin is also used to lower high blood sugars. This High Blood Sugar Regular is used to bring down high blood sugars more quickly. Less damage is likely when blood sugars are high for shorter periods of time.

But caution is needed in lowering high blood sugars so as not to cause unwanted lows. For safety, you need to know how many points your blood sugar drops on each unit of Regular. Once you know your own sensitivity to Regular, you can set up a personalized table that gives the number of units to take for highs before or after meals. This table is sometimes referred to as a sliding scale.

This chapter shows:

- How to determine how far your blood sugar will drop on each unit of Regular
- How much High Blood Sugar Regular to add to the Carb Regular for premeal highs
- How much High Blood Sugar Regular to take for high blood sugars between meals

To set up your own High Blood Sugar Regular scale, you will need to select safe and reasonable target goals for both before and after meals. This goal setting is always done with help from your physician/health care team. Since your blood sugar naturally rises after eating, the target goal after a meal is higher than before a meal. For instance, a target of 100 mg/dl (5.6 mmol) before eating and 180 mg/dl (10 mmol) two to three hours after eating is reasonable for many people on flexible insulin therapy.

Your own targets should be discussed with your physician/health care team and tailored to your special needs. In pregnancy, lower target blood sugars are required, while someone with a history of hypoglycemia unawareness will need higher targets. For high blood sugars at bedtime, a good rule of thumb is to take half the usual dose of High Blood Sugar Regular.

THE 1500 RULE

A great tool for setting up a personalized scale was developed by Paul C. Davidson, M.D., Medical Director of the Diabetes Treatment Center at HCA West Paces Ferry Hospital in Atlanta.[44] His "1500 Rule" states that someone's blood sugar drop on a unit of Regular can be closely estimated by dividing how much total insulin they use a day into the number 1500 (80 works well in the mmol system).

How many points the blood sugar drops on each unit of Regular depends on weight and on sensitivity to insulin. Weight and sensitivity to insulin determine the total amount of insulin needed each day. For instance, someone using only 20 units of insulin a day is usually thin and quite sensitive to insulin. (An exception is someone with Type II diabetes who is resistant to insulin, but requires only 20 units a day to supplement their own insulin production.)

High Blood Sugar Regular For Highs BEFORE Meals								
Total daily units of insulin =	20	25	30	40	50	60	75	100
Expected drop in sugar per unit of Regular =	75	60	50	38	33	25	20	15
Extra Regular needed before meals =								
B 100	0	0	0	0	0	0	0	0
L 140	0	0	0	1	1	1	2	2
O 180	1	1	1	2	2	3	4	5
O 220	1	2	2	3	4	4	6	8
D 260*	2	2	3	4	5	6	8	10
S 300*	2	3	4	5	6	8	10	13
U 340*	3	4	4	6	8	9	12	16
G 380*	3	4	5	7	9	11	14	18
A 420*	4	5	6	8	10	12	16	21
R * check urine for ketones								

Table 16.1 High Blood Sugar Regular Scales for Different People

Their blood sugar will drop farther on one unit of Regular—usually around 75 points (4.2 mmol)—than someone who uses 75 units of insulin a day. The second person on 75 units will have their blood sugar drop about 20 points (1.1 mmol) per unit of Regular.

A SAMPLE HIGH BLOOD SUGAR SCALE

A personalized High Blood Sugar Regular Sliding Scale can be set up using the information in Table 16.1. How much Regular insulin to take for a high blood sugar is determined by how far this blood sugar is above a selected target and by how many points that person's blood sugar will drop on each unit of Regular.

Table 16.2 shows one sample High Blood Sugar Regular Scale for someone who weighs 160 pounds and has good control using 38 units of insulin a day. The scale was created by referring to Table 13.1 to determine that this person's blood sugar was likely to drop about 40 points for each unit of Regular. The target blood sugars were chosen with his physician's help as 100 mg/dl (5.6 mmol) before a meal and 180 mg/dl (10 mmol) two to three hours after a meal. This sample scale gives the dose of Regular, in half unit increments, that this person needs for high blood sugars that might occur before or after meals. (When precise doses are desired, half unit increments can be given with a 30 unit syringe.)

For premeal highs, this extra Regular can be added to the Carb Regular given for the food in the meal. You would not use extra High Blood Sugar Regular, of course, if your blood sugars fall from high readings to normal on their own. Another situation where you might not need this extra insulin is if you plan to exercise after the meal.

With experience, you will also discover when you need extra Regular for high blood sugars that occur between meals. In some situations, such as when Regular was taken just before eating a food with a high glycemic index, a reading of 200 or 300 mg/dl (11.1 to 16.7 mmol) might be ignored because the blood sugar will return to normal as the Regular begins to take effect.

In other circumstances, however, a blood sugar of 200 or 300 mg/dl following a meal will not drop to normal unless extra insulin is taken. It is important to understand what your own blood sugars do, and to have an individualized High Blood Sugar Regular Table to guide you in taking the correct dose. Get personal guidance for this from your physician/health care team.

How far the blood sugar drops on a unit of Regular generally stays the same unless infection, ketoacidosis, a marked change in physical activity, or other complicating factors are present. If your blood sugar drop per unit of Regular varies greatly from one time of day to another, be sure you are counting carbohydrates accurately, then retest the long-acting insulin to make sure it has been accurately set.

TESTING HIGH BLOOD SUGAR REGULAR DOSES

The starting doses of Regular for high blood sugars that you determined in previous chapters are only estimates. They have to be tested to see if they will work for you. Determine your own sliding scale by estimating a starting point drop per unit of Regular with your physician's help, and then test it and adjust as needed from the test results.

The flow chart in Figure 16.3 on the next page shows how to test High Blood Sugar Regular Doses. Select first, with your physician's help, your target blood sugar before meals. This is usually 90 to 140 mg/dl (5 to 7.8 mmol) for testing purposes. The test can then be carried out whenever a blood sugar is above 200 mg/dl (11.1 mmol) at least five hours after the last dose of Regular insulin was given, and three hours after the last food was eaten. Eating has to be delayed for another five hours to complete the test.

High Blood Sugar Regular Sliding Scale		
Blood Sugar Reading (mg/dl)	Units Of Regular Needed For A High Blood Sugar	
	Before Meals	After Meals
100-119	0	0
120-139	0.5 unit	0
140-159	1.0 unit	0
160-179	1.5 units	0
180-199	2.0 units	0
200-219	2.5 units	0.5 unit
220-239	3.0 units	1.0 unit
240-259	3.5 units	1.5 units
260-279	4.0 units	2.0 units
280-299	4.5 units	2.5 units
300-319	5.0 units	3.0 units
320-339	5.5 units	3.5 units
340-359	6.0 units	4.0 units
360-379	6.5 units	4.5 units
380-399	7.0 units	5.0 units

Table 16.2 Sample Scale for 160 pound person using 38 units of Insulin a day

This test is repeated until a ratio is found that brings your blood sugar to close to normal on two consecutive tests. An ideal ratio brings high blood sugars to within 30 points of your target blood sugar four to five hours after the insulin is taken. Test the blood sugar often during the test to prevent a low blood sugar.

After successful testing, you can create your own personalized High Blood Sugar Regular Scale using the form at the back of this book. The High Blood Sugar Regular Scale is one of the most important tools for helping you fine tune your blood sugar control. When combined with correct doses of long-acting insulin and Carb Regular, the ability to lower high blood sugars safely is the last major piece of information needed for excellent control.

However, you will see in the next chapter that you must also take into account the amount of unused Regular insulin that is present due to recent doses of Regular.

Table 16.3 How to Test Your High Blood Sugar Regular

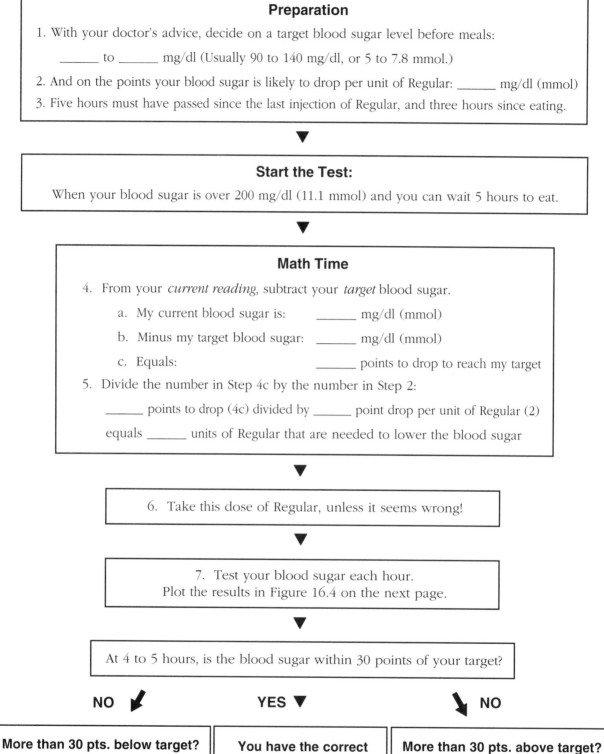

Preparation

1. With your doctor's advice, decide on a target blood sugar level before meals:

    _____ to _____ mg/dl (Usually 90 to 140 mg/dl, or 5 to 7.8 mmol.)

2. And on the points your blood sugar is likely to drop per unit of Regular: _____ mg/dl (mmol)

3. Five hours must have passed since the last injection of Regular, and three hours since eating.

▼

Start the Test:

When your blood sugar is over 200 mg/dl (11.1 mmol) and you can wait 5 hours to eat.

▼

Math Time

4. From your *current reading*, subtract your *target* blood sugar.

    a. My current blood sugar is: _____ mg/dl (mmol)

    b. Minus my target blood sugar: _____ mg/dl (mmol)

    c. Equals: _____ points to drop to reach my target

5. Divide the number in Step 4c by the number in Step 2:

    _____ points to drop (4c) divided by _____ point drop per unit of Regular (2)

    equals _____ units of Regular that are needed to lower the blood sugar

▼

6. Take this dose of Regular, unless it seems wrong!

▼

7. Test your blood sugar each hour.
Plot the results in Figure 16.4 on the next page.

▼

At 4 to 5 hours, is the blood sugar within 30 points of your target?

NO ↙   **YES** ▼   ↘ **NO**

More than 30 pts. below target?	**You have the correct ratio of points dropped per unit of Regular. Retest to verify.**	**More than 30 pts. above target?**
Retest using a larger point drop number (i.e., if it was 1R/35 pts., use 1R/38 pts.)		Retest using a smaller point drop number (i.e., if it was 1R/35 pts., use 1R/32 pts.)

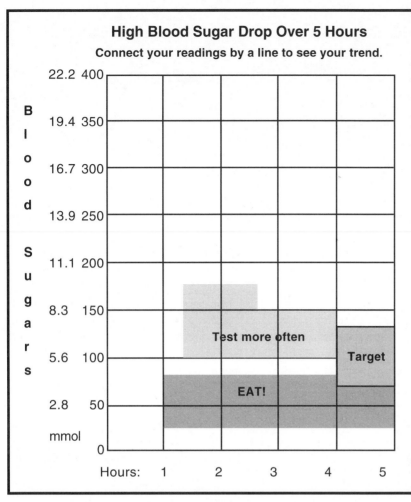

High Blood Sugar Drop Over 5 Hours

Connect your readings by a line to see your trend.

Figure 16.4 See Directions At Right

Record Your Blood Sugar Each Hour On The Graph.

As you test your blood sugars in Step 7 of Figure 16.3, plot your results on the graph to the left (Figure 16.4).

Be sure to test more often if you see your plotted line going down to the left of the target zone!

TIPS ON HIGH BLOOD SUGAR REGULAR

- The correct ratio of Regular to number of points (mg/dl or mmol) the blood sugar will drop brings a high blood sugar to within 30 points of the Target Blood Sugar 5 hours after the dose was given.

- The need for Regular insulin changes when ketoacidosis, an infection, a change in weight, or a change in physical activity occur. Test more often when giving doses of Regular for high blood sugars in these special circumstances.

- If an unexpected high blood sugar occurs, try to determine why this is happening.

- Signs of an incorrect ratio for the High Blood Sugar Regular:
    Too little insulin: the blood sugar does not drop to your target as expected
    Too much insulin: the blood sugar often drops below your target or drops sooner than expected.

- If High Blood Sugar Regular is required frequently, either the background insulin doses or the doses for Carb Regular are too low.

- *Quick Regular Check:* Do your doses of Regular for the day make up 40 percent to 55 percent of your total daily insulin dose?

Never argue with a doctor; he has inside information.
Bob and Ray

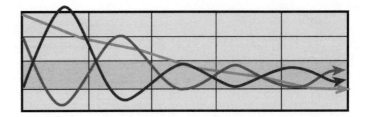

The Unused Insulin Rule

17

A big advantage of flexible insulin therapy comes from giving frequent doses of insulin as the need arises. Regular can be given for dinner, more for the unplanned dessert, then another dose for the high blood sugar later. But a problem surfaces as these injections of Regular begin to overlap. How much of the previous Regular is still working? After several injections, the bedtime blood sugar has to be interpreted in the light of all the insulin given earlier in the evening that has yet to work. A normal blood sugar at bedtime could be dangerous if you forgot the large residual dose of Regular insulin still working.

This chapter helps you determine how much insulin or carbohydrate you need once you've checked your bedtime blood sugar. It also guides you through situations where two or more injections have been given within the last four to five hours.

This chapter:

- Explains the Unused Insulin Rule
- Shows how the Unused Insulin Tables work
- Tells you how to resolve differences between the Unused Insulin Rule and the High Blood Sugar Regular Sliding Scale covered in the last chapter

What Is The Unused Insulin Rule?

The Unused Insulin Rule is a way to estimate how many units of Regular insulin are still working from recent injections. It helps in deciding whether more insulin or more carbohydrate is needed at any time of the day. Most people find that an injection of Regular starts working a half hour after the injection, peaks two to three hours later, and stops dropping the blood sugar after five to six hours. From this timetable of action we get the Unused Insulin Rule:

After an injection of Regular, 16% to 20% of it will be used each hour.

This rule lets you determine how much Regular is left to work from earlier injections. The 20 percent-per-hour guide works for those who are more sensitive to insulin. If you are younger and rarely take more than 10 units in an injection, you will likely find little effect from Regular insulin four to five hours after an injection. Insulin works longer in some people, however, and if you are older or take larger doses, you may find your insulin is still lowering the blood sugar at six to seven hours. If so, you will want to use the 16 percent per hour guide.

UNUSED INSULIN

Tables 17.1 and 17.2 interpret the Unused Insulin Rule into practical terms. Table 17.1 (20 percent per hour) shows how much insulin per hour is left from an injection in those who get a faster response from their Regular insulin. Table 17.2 (16 percent per hour) on the next page shows how much insulin per hour is left from an injection in those who get a slower response from their insulin. Use the table that you and your physician feel is most appropriate.

Example One: Let's say your blood sugar was off the scale of your meter (somewhere above 450 mg/dl or 25 mmol), your ketones were negative, and you took 8 units of Regular to bring the high reading down. You check your blood sugar again three

Faster Insulin Table—20% per hour

Amount In Original Injection	Units Of Regular Insulin Left After:				
	1 Hour	2 Hours	3 Hours	4 Hours	5 Hours
1 unit	0.8	0.6	0.4	0.2	0
2 units	1.6	1.2	0.8	0.4	0
3 units	2.4	1.8	1.2	0.6	0
4 units	3.2	2.4	1.6	0.8	0
5 units	4.0	3.0	2.0	1.0	0
6 units	4.8	3.6	2.4	1.2	0
7 units	5.6	4.2	2.8	1.4	0
8 units	6.4	4.8	3.2	1.6	0
9 units	7.2	5.4	3.6	1.8	0
10 units	8.0	6.0	4.0	2.0	0

Table 17.1 Use this table if you get a quicker action from Regular insulin

hours later and find it now measures 300 mg/dl (16.7 mmol). Should you take more Regular? To find out, let's use Table 17.1 because you are fairly sensitive to insulin. Using this table, you find that in 3 hours, 20 percent X 3 hours or 60 percent of your Regular is gone. You took 8 units, so 8 units X .60 = 4.8 units have been used. That means that 8 units minus 4.8 units or 3.2 units of Regular are left to work. (See Table 17.1 for confirmation.)

Let's say that your blood sugar drops 38 points on 1 unit of Regular. You can then calculate the remaining activity of the earlier injection as follows:

3.2 units left times 38 points dropped per unit equals 122 points
Your blood sugar is still likely to drop 122 points from the previous injection.

Since your blood sugar is 300, you can expect to be at 300 - 122 = 178 in two more hours when the remainder of the 8 units of Regular has been used. You now know you're likely to need more insulin if you want to lower your blood sugar to 100. You can then estimate how much more Regular insulin is likely to be needed:

178 minus 100 equals 78 more points to drop
78 points divided by 38 points per units equals
2.0 more units needed to bring the blood sugar down.

Of course, these calculations depend on already being on flexible insulin therapy and having set up your long-acting insulin doses correctly. Test your blood sugar more frequently when using the Unused Insulin Rule. To avoid nighttime insulin reactions, don't use as much extra Regular for highs at bedtime without your physician/health care team's advice. If they advise taking the full dose, set your alarm to wake you in 2 or 3 hours to test again and thereby avoid a low.

By using the Unused Insulin Rule and your knowledge of how far your blood sugar drops on each unit of Regular, you are able to determine:

1. How much insulin is still left to work from previous injections

2. How much additional Regular is needed to lower a high blood sugar

3. Whether too much insulin may already have been given

Example Two: As another example, let's say you go out for breakfast to a new restaurant. You order pancakes and fruit, but don't take your Regular until your food arrives because you're not sure how many carbohydrates it will have. When your plate arrives, you estimate you'll need 7 units for breakfast and then take your injection of Regular. Two hours later when you measure your blood sugar, you find it's 200 mg/dl (11.1 mmol). You've previously found that your blood sugar drops 40 points on each unit of Regular. Do you need to take an injection of Regular to lower this blood sugar?

To answer this question, let's assume you get a slower and longer action from your Regular insulin. You took 7 units of Regular two hours ago. After two hours 32 percent (16 percent times 2 hours) of it has been used. This leaves 68 percent of this last injection still left to work, and from Table 17.2:

Slower Insulin Table—16% per hour

Amount In Original Injection	Units Of Regular Insulin Left After:					
	1 Hour	2 Hours	3 Hours	4 Hours	5 Hours	6 Hours
1 unit	0.8	0.7	0.5	0.3	0.2	0
2 units	1.7	1.3	1.0	0.7	0.3	0
3 units	2.5	2.0	1.5	1.0	0.5	0
4 units	3.3	2.7	2.0	1.3	0.7	0
5 units	4.2	3.3	2.5	1.7	0.8	0
6 units	5.0	4.0	3.0	2.0	1.0	0
7 units	5.8	4.7	3.5	2.3	1.2	0
8 units	6.7	5.3	4.0	2.7	1.3	0
9 units	7.5	6.0	4.5	3.0	1.5	0
10 units	8.3	6.7	5.0	3.3	1.7	0

Table 17.2 Use this table if you get a slower action from Regular insulin

7 units times 0.68 equals *4.7 units still active.*

So, as the Regular continues to work over the next 4 hours, your blood sugar should drop an additional:

40 points dropped per unit times 4.7 units left equals *188 points*

At that time your blood sugar will be:

200 minus 188 points still to drop equals *12 (predicted blood sugar).*

It appears that not only is an injection of Regular not needed, but you may need extra carbohydrate in the next hour or two to prevent a low. A followup blood sugar in 60 to 90 minutes will clarify this. Skip the injection, and eat extra carbohydrate if your blood sugar requires this.

RESOLVING DIFFERENCES BETWEEN THE UI RULE AND THE HBSR SCALE

As you may have noticed in the last example, discrepancies can occur when estimating how much insulin is needed when you use two different methods: the Unused Insulin Rule described in this chapter and the High Blood Sugar Regular Scale determined in Chapter 16.

Suppose you had used the High Blood Sugar Regular Scale in Example Two when you had a blood sugar of 200 mg/dl (11.1 mmol) two hours after eating. You might have calculated:

200 minus 160 (your target blood sugar after eating) equals 40 more points to drop
40 points to drop divided by 40 points dropped per unit equals *1 unit of insulin still needed*

Using your High Blood Sugar Regular Scale, you might take an extra unit of Regular in this situation. However, according to the Unused Insulin Rule you really need more carbohydrate to prevent a low blood sugar. This discrepancy between the two rules comes from having taken the injection just before eating. You can't take an injection just before eating and expect a post-meal reading of 160 mg/dl (8.9 mmol)! This example shows that rules are never perfect. Rules only provide guidance. More important is to base your decisions upon your own judgment and experience, guided by the advice of your physician/health care team.

Tip: In the situation above, taking the breakfast injection so close to the meal allowed the blood sugar to rise more than it would have otherwise. In situations where you plan to eat at a new restaurant, you can take a partial dose of Regular to lead the meal, then catch up on the remainder of the dose once you see the plate. Two hours after the injection is also a relatively short time to get a true reading of how well the Carb Regular covered that meal. A blood sugar taken three hours after the injection could give more information in this situation.

The Unused Insulin Rule is more conservative than the High Blood Sugar Regular Scale. That is, the Unused Insulin Rule is more likely to overestimate how much the blood sugar will drop and underestimate how much additional Regular may be needed. It is intended to be conservative in order to avoid insulin reactions caused by chasing high blood sugars with too much insulin.

When there is a conflict between a dose of Regular recommended by the Unused Insulin Rule and one recommended by your High Blood Sugar Regular Scale, decide on a dose only after weighing all the factors that may affect your blood sugar. When in doubt, always use the smaller dose.

Caution: It's not wise to take Regular more often than every two or three hours. At least three hours are needed to get an idea of what the last injection is doing. Taking Regular more often than this allows too much insulin activity to build up, complicates your computations, and makes an insulin reaction likely. New, faster insulins like Lispro, which is expected to be available in 1996, could be given every two hours with less risk of insulin buildup.

*Opportunity is missed by most people
because it is dressed in overalls and looks like work.*

Thomas Edison

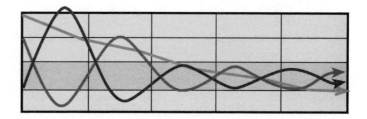

WHEN TO CHANGE THE LONG-ACTING INSULIN

18

Long-acting insulin doses are not changed unless there's a clear reason to do so. But some situations demand that the long-acting insulin (including the Regular insulin in some of these situations) be changed. Part of a comprehensive flexible insulin program is knowing when to make these changes. In this chapter, you will learn about some of the things that make these changes necessary.

CHANGE IN ACTIVITY

Physical fitness determines much of our sensitivity to insulin. Marathon runners, for example, are quite sensitive and have half as much insulin circulating in the blood as a person of the same height and weight who doesn't exercise heavily. Whenever there's a substantial increase in the level of activity, a reduction in the long-acting insulin is almost always required. If you work as a moderately active flight attendant but are going to spend two weeks on a bicycling trip, plan on lowering your long-acting insulin doses.

Extra muscle activity and improved muscle tone brought about by activities like long-distance bicycling can greatly increase sensitivity to insulin. Long, intense activities like this may require that insulin doses be rapidly lowered. As much as a 30 percent to 40 percent reduction in the background insulin dose may be needed at the start of such strenuous activity. Always plan ahead for major changes in your activity level. A quick call to your physician/health care team can prevent major problems here.

Just the opposite happens when the activity level is lowered. If you had been working as a framer on a construction crew, but now work at a desk as a project cost estimator, this decrease in activity is likely to increase your need for long-acting insulin.

When exercise lasts less than 60 minutes, a reduction in the long-acting insulin is usually not needed. But for moderate or strenuous exercise that lasts longer than 60 to 90 minutes, a lowering of the longer-acting insulin may be necessary.

CHANGE IN WEIGHT

Your bathroom scale is a barometer of your insulin doses. When you weigh more, you need more long-acting (and Regular) insulin. As your weight drops, your long-acting insulin has to be lowered. Two things play a role in how you change your long-acting insulin during weight changes.

Setting Your Insulin Doses

First is the speed of the weight change. If swimsuit season is suddenly upon you, or you decide at the last moment to attend your high school reunion, or out-of-town relatives call to tell you they'll be visiting next month, weight panic often sets in. Where did those extra pounds come from and how can they be shed quickly? Eating may be quickly reduced in this concern over image. Although losing weight in this way is not recommended, it is sometimes done.

Any fast weight loss requires a quick reduction in the long-acting insulin. A reduction of 10 to 30 percent may be needed at the start of a restricted calorie intake. Regular insulin, of course, is also lowered in relation to the drop in carbohydrate intake and to the increased sensitivity to insulin that occurs with weight loss.

The second thing to be considered is how much weight is lost or gained. A gradual change of five pounds or so may have little effect on the long-acting insulin doses. If the shift is 10 pounds or more, an adjustment in these doses will very likely be needed. The greater the weight change and the faster the weight change, the more you need to change your long-acting insulin.

GASTROPARESIS

Gastroparesis is damage to the nerves that control the wavelike motion of the intestines. This loss of normal intestinal motion can cause food to be absorbed more slowly after a meal than normal, creating problems in blood sugar control because of this delay. When a person with gastroparesis takes Regular to cover food, an insulin reaction often occurs two to three hours later. This may be followed by a high blood sugar some six or eight hours later as the meal begins to be converted to glucose in the blood. A person with gastroparesis may benefit from a higher than normal dose of long-acting insulin in the morning to cover eating, with little or no Regular for meals.

Most blood sugar problems have nothing to do with gastroparesis. Never blame your own control problems on gastroparesis without adequate testing and a thorough discussion with your physician. Be aware that there are also effective medicines that can improve this problem. Discuss this with your physician.

ILLNESSES

Illnesses, especially bacterial infections, place extra stress on the body. Extra Regular and long-acting insulin is often needed to fight this physical stress. During bacterial illnesses, like pneumonia, a strep throat, an impacted wisdom tooth, a bladder infection, or a sinus infection, more insulin is needed. The need is especially acute when the illness is accompanied by a fever. Bacteria are usually more stressful to the body than viruses and can easily cause the total insulin need to double. After an antibiotic has been started, however, any temporary increase in insulin doses has to be quickly lowered to prevent insulin reactions.

Illnesses that last several weeks, like hepatitis and mononucleosis, often require an increase in the long-acting insulin doses. Shorter viral illnesses, like a cold or flu, have more varied effects on blood sugars. It is often easier to control blood sugars during short-term viral illnesses by using High Blood Sugar Regular as needed, rather than by raising the long-acting insulin. Extra Regular may be needed even though eating is reduced. Always remember:

The quickest way to lower an occasional high blood sugar is to take Regular and NOT a long-acting insulin.

However, if blood sugars are often high, raising the long-acting insulin may be best.

More insulin can be given quickly with Regular than by increasing the long-acting insulin. An injection of 10 units of Regular begins to work in 30 to 60 minutes and will have completed its work in lowering the blood sugar in five to six hours. Ten units of Lente or NPH does not begin to work for three or four hours and will not complete its action until the next day. The extra speed in insulin delivery from Regular can be critical during an illness. Injections of Regular can also be repeated every few hours as needed (see Chapters 16 and 17).

Illnesses that cause vomiting or diarrhea may mean you can't eat, but they do not affect the background insulin need. Less eating can usually be offset by taking less Regular. However, if Regular has been taken for a meal, but one is unable to eat or vomiting occurs, carbohydrate has to be taken in. Apple juice, regular 7-UP®, honey dissolved inside the cheek, or other quick sugar has to be consumed. Be certain to test your blood sugars often or have someone else test it for you during any illness.

MENSES

Many women find their blood sugar rises in the days just before their period begins. Sometimes this increase is small enough that it does not require changing the long-acting insulin doses. Many women, however, find they need a substantial increase in both Regular and long-acting insulins during the few days prior to their period. This extra need for insulin quickly returns to baseline on the first day of the period.

Once a change in insulin requirement during menses has been determined and blood sugars are stabilized, the timing of monthly periods and the increased need for insulin becomes more predictable. This change in insulin doses can be anticipated at about the same time during future cycles. If you observe a monthly change occurring, discuss it with your physician/health care team for a way to match it with a cyclic insulin adjustment. By maintaining the blood sugars close to normal during the premenstrual rise, both symptoms and control are improved.

MEDICATIONS

Certain drugs increase the need for insulin. Primary among these are steroids or glucocorticoids like prednisone and cortisone. Whether taken for poison ivy, for illnesses such as lupus or asthma, or as an injection into an inflamed joint, steroids generally raise insulin need sharply. John Walsh got a severe case of poison oak while clearing fire brush out of a field. (Never use a weed whacker on poison oak!) This required taking prednisone tablets for a few days and caused a marked rise in blood sugars and insulin requirements. Insulin doses were raised, at times to levels four times those normally used.

Occasionally, the physician who properly recommends the use of oral or injected steroids for medical problems may be unaware how dramatically they can affect blood sugar levels. Steroids injected into joints will usually increase insulin need for three to five days. If steroids are required, make sure the physician prescribing them is aware of your diabetes.

Contact your physician/health care team as soon as possible to discuss the extra insulin that is likely to be needed. Be prepared to test more frequently to compensate for increased and decreased insulin need. It's a good idea when any new medication is prescribed to make sure the physician knows you have diabetes and to ask how it might affect your blood sugar.

POST-MEAL SPIKES

Many people notice that a couple of hours after eating, their blood sugars rise to very high levels. If the blood sugar remains high until the next meal, the solution is usually simple: either raise the Carb Regular taken for that meal the next time it is eaten or lower the amount of carbohydrate in it. However, when the blood sugar spikes above a desired range (usually 150 to 180 mg/dl, or 8.3 to 10 mmol) between meals and then returns to normal before the next meal, a more complicated problem exists. The Carb Regular can't be raised or a low blood sugar will occur.

A common cause of spiking between meals is taking the Carb Regular too close to the meal. Try taking it earlier before the meal if this is the cause. If Regular was taken 30 to 45 minutes before eating and the food choices are good, raise the long-acting insulin dose and maintian or slightly lower the Carb Regular. This combination can often reduce post-meal spikes. Usually only a small increase in the long-acting insulin dose is needed, about one or two units or 10 percent of the long-acting insulin dose. Discuss this with your physician\health care team.

THYROID DISEASE

Thyroid disease is both more common than diabetes and more common with diabetes. Women are especially at risk for thyroid disease. Hashimoto's thyroiditis (an inflamed condition of the thyroid first discovered by a Japanese surgeon named Hakura Hashimoto) is the most common cause of thyroid disorders. It is especially common in Type I diabetes because both disorders are an autoimmune attack on a hormone producing gland. But those with Type II diabetes are not immune. Thyroid failures becomes more common as we age. Almost one out of every 10 women over the age of 65 has a low thyroid condition, mostly due to Hashimoto's.

Because thyroid disease develops gradually over a period of weeks to months, it often creates problems in control long before the cause is identified. Both an overactive and an underactive thyroid will lead to control problems. Hashimoto's is an attack by the immune system on the thyroid where thyroid hormone is stored, and excess thyroid hormone may be released into the blood in its early stages. The resulting increased metabolism indirectly causes blood sugars to rise and requires that insulin doses be raised. Not everyone goes through this increased metabolism phase. Some people go straight to the lower thyroid phase.

As the disease continues over several months, less and less thyroid hormone is released, and many people become hypothyroid or low thyroid. Suddenly, the person who was hyperthyroid is now hypothyroid and begins to have unexpected low blood sugars and insulin doses have to be lowered. So, if you are finding that your insulin doses have unexpectedly changed and you have thyroid symptoms like excess nervousness, tiredness, or problems sleeping, discuss this with your physician. And, remember, if you start on a thyroid medication, your insulin doses will likely need to be bumped up again.

ENVIRONMENTAL CHANGES

Changes in your external environment may also require a change in insulin dosage. As temperatures change outside a home, the thermostat in the home's heating/air conditioning system responds by raising or lowering the temperature. As your utility bill will tell you, maintaining a constant temperature can require lots of energy. Your body acts the same way, using more glucose and fat as it warms or cools itself. The increased metabolic rate required to cool or heat the body uses additional energy that may lower the blood sugar. If you are outside in unusually hot or cold weather, some reduction in insulin doses may be needed. This is especially true in hot weather when the body uses more energy in cooling and sends more blood flow to the skin. The increased circulation picks up insulin faster from the injection site and speeds up the action of insulin. A lower background insulin dose may be needed.

A similar circumstance happens when you move to higher altitudes. More energy is needed to breath and pump blood as the air becomes thinner. The resulting increase in metabolism is especially apparent in the first few days after arriving at a higher elevation. Until the body acclimates, less long-acting insulin or extra carbohydrate may be required.

The older I get, the better I was.
T-shirt slogan

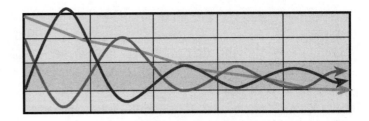

INSULIN REACTIONS:
RECOGNIZING, TREATING AND PREVENTING

19

Insulin reactions are of concern to most people who use insulin. Mild reactions can be annoying and embarrassing, while a severe reaction can be dangerous. During a reaction, you may shake, sweat and feel disoriented. Or you may feel relatively normal, although others around you may notice distinct differences. Thinking and coordination deteriorate as the blood sugar drops. Loss of coordination, release of stress hormones, and irritability usually start when the blood sugar goes below 55 or 60 (3.1 to 3.3 mmol), although these changes are not always apparent to the person having the reaction. Regardless of how well you feel or think you feel, a blood sugar below 60 mg/dl is an insulin reaction and carries with it some danger.

This chapter discusses the following aspects of insulin reactions:

- Causes
- Symptoms
- Treatment
- Prevention

CAUSES OF INSULIN REACTIONS

Reactions are most likely to happen:

1. When too much insulin is taken
2. When insulin is taken for a meal, but the meal is missed, delayed or interrupted
3. When large or frequent doses of Regular are used to bring down highs
4. After drinking alcohol
5. During and after exercise

Too Much Insulin

When a person first changes to multiple injections with flexible insulin therapy, the insulin doses are often set too high. As a person switches to better use of insulin, less insulin is often needed. During this transition period, insulin reactions are more likely.

This extra vulnerability may also be increased by the natural enthusiasm, experimentation and uncertainty that accompanies the use of flexible insulin therapy. For the first time you have the ability to maintain normal blood sugars. This feeling is positive and can help in the goal of keeping blood sugars between 70 to 120 mg/dl (3.9 to 6.7 mmol) before meals and no higher than 140 to 180 mg/dl (7.8 to 10 mmol) after meals. Be willing, however, to set realistic intermediate goals, to pace yourself, and to celebrate small steps as you move toward a normal range.

Most important, check your blood sugar often. As your physician/health care team gives you more responsibility in adjusting your insulin doses, do so only with adequate testing. Adjust insulin doses gradually and in agreement with your physician/health care team's recommendations.

SYMPTOMS OF INSULIN REACTIONS

Insulin reactions can occur without symptoms, with minor symptoms, or with full blown symptoms. Symptoms vary from person to person, and from reaction to reaction. A reaction may first be recognized by the person having the reaction, or by others around them.

In Table 19.1, you see common symptoms of insulin reactions. Recognizing that an insulin reaction is underway allows early treatment. Symptoms for insulin reactions may become more subtle when using flexible insulin therapy. With three or more injections, people often find that blood sugars drop more slowly than with one or two larger injections. This slower blood sugar drop provides more time to respond to a low blood sugar, but it can also cause fewer symptoms. Learn to recognize the more subtle symptoms.

One or more of these symptoms can occur during any reaction; some may never occur. Check your blood sugar whenever a low blood sugar is suspected by you or by someone else. If someone else asks you to check your blood sugar, do so. Blood sugar testing will alert you to insulin reactions you may be having with minimal symptoms or with minimal awareness of your symptoms. The faster you recognize a reaction, the faster you can respond and return to a normal blood sugar.

Insulin Reaction Symptoms
Sweating
Shaking
Iirritability
Blurred vision
Fast heart rate
Sudden tiredness
Dizziness and confusion
Numbness of the lips
Nausea or vomiting
Frequent sighing
Headache
Silliness
Tingling

Table 19.1 You may experience many of these symptoms

Nighttime Reactions

Symptoms for nighttime reactions can be particularly hard to recognize, especially if they start during sleep. If you wake up during the night with any of the symptoms below, check your blood sugar immediately. Or eat quick-acting carbohydrate and then check.

These symptoms include:

- Nightmares
- Waking up very alert or with a fast heart rate
- Damp night clothes, sheets or pillow
- Restlessness and inability to go back to sleep

Or you may have waking symptoms of a nighttime reaction listed below:

- Waking up with a headache or "foggy headed"
- Unusually high blood sugar after breakfast or before lunch
- A small amount of ketones but no glucose in the morning urine
- Loss of memory for words or names

If you have any of the nighttime symptoms, testing a 2 a.m. blood sugar for a few nights can do wonders in identifying and correcting this problem. Review possible causes and take action to avoid a reoccurrence.

TREATMENT OF INSULIN REACTIONS

The First Rule of Good Control: *Stop the LOWS first!*

With frequent or severe reactions, a major correction is needed.
A reduction of at least 10 percent in the total daily insulin dose is usually required.

Keep in mind that one insulin reaction increases the risk for another. Researchers in Virginia found that the chances for having a second insulin reaction after an initial reaction are greatly increased: 46 percent in the next 24 hours, 24 percent on the second day, and 12 percent on the third day after the original reaction.[45] Not only is the risk higher, but symptoms of the low blood sugar during the second reaction are harder to recognize.

Treat Reactions Quickly

Not even the most conscientious person can prevent every reaction. When a reaction does occur, the next best step is to relieve symptoms quickly.

The best treatment for lows is often a combination of simple and complex carbohydrates, plus some protein. Ten to fifteen grams of simple carbohydrates, such as glucose, Sweet Tarts® or honey, will quickly raise the blood sugar 30 to 75 points under most circumstances.

Treating your insulin reactions with quick carbs returns your blood sugar to normal faster than eating or drinking anything else. Raising the low blood sugar quickly helps shut off the release of stress hormones. This lowers the chance of having a high blood sugar afterward and improves your chances of recognizing the next reaction. You'll feel better if the body is quickly resupplied with the fuel it needs. Your brain, muscles and other cells will thank you.

Glucose (also called dextrose) is the "sugar" in "blood sugar." Glucose also comes in tablets or tubes and can also be obtained in several candies like Sweet Tarts® (see Table 19.3). Sweet Tarts are good because they quickly break down as 100 percent glucose in the blood, and are an excellent choice for raising blood sugars. Maltose, which is made of two glucose molecules, is also quite fast. Both maltose and honey are fast, but messy. Table sugar, however, is made from one glucose molecule and one fructose molecule. When table sugar breaks down

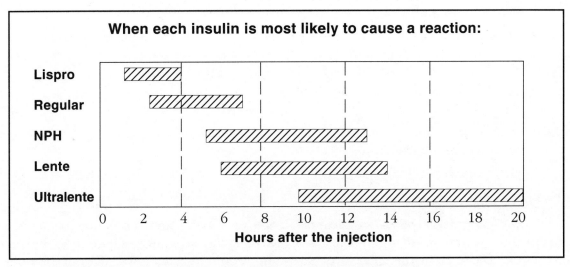

Fig. 19.2 Different insulins have different peak action times

in the stomach, only 50 percent of it is immediately available as glucose. Fruit juices, like orange juice, contain mostly fructose and are a poor choice for reactions because they take so long to raise the blood sugar. See the glycemic index in Appendix B at the back of this book for more guidance.

How much glucose is needed? A good rule of thumb is that 1 gram of glucose raises the blood sugar 3, 4, or 5 points (for weights of 200 lb., 150 lb., and 100 lb., respectively). A 5 gram glucose tablet should raise the blood sugar between 15 and 25 points, depending on your weight and acitvity.

Use 15 to 20 grams of quick carbohydrate for all low blood sugars. Table 19.3 lists a variety of these. Each contains 15 grams of glucose or an equivalent sugar, and should rapidly raise the blood sugar between 45 and 75 points for people who weigh between 200 lb. and 100 lb., respectively. Test your blood sugar again in 20 to 30 minutes to ensure the low has been corrected.

Check to see how many grams of carbohydrate are in each glucose tablet you use to make sure you actually get 15 to 20 grams.

Remember that thinking and coordination remain abnormal for 30 minutes after the blood sugar has been brought back to normal. Wait 30 to 45 minutes after the blood sugar has returned to normal before driving a car or operating machinery.

Once you've eaten simple carbs to quickly raise the blood sugar, consider the situation again. A recent injection of Regular, extra exercise, or a missed meal all demand that more than 10 or 15 grams of glucose be taken. At bedtime, in particular, have an extra 10 grams or so of carbohydrate, such as a glass of milk or half an apple. Raw cornstarch is a complex carbohydrate that breaks down very slowly, and seems

Quick Carbs To Keep On Hand
Each of these has 15 grams of quick carbs:
1 tablespoon of honey
3 BD Glucose Tablets
3 Smartie® Rolls (3" cellophane rolls)
4 CanAm Dex4® Glucose Tablets
5 Dextrosols®
5 Wacky Wafers®
6 SweetTart® packets (3 tabs/packet)
7 Pixy Stix
8 Sweet Tarts® (3/4" Lifesaver size)
14 Smarties® (3/4" diameter roll)

Table 19.3 Glucose comes in many forms

to help in preventing overnight lows. An alternative is to have a high protein food, like cheese or peanut butter. Both proteins and complex carbohydrates keep the blood sugar from dropping for some time.

Treatment Plan For Typical Insulin Reactions

1. Eat 15 to 20 grams of quick-acting carbohydrates (Table 19.3).

2. Consider how long it is to your next meal and whether additional complex carbohydrates with protein are needed (crackers and cheese or peanut butter, half an apple with cheese, or a cup of milk).

3. Test the blood sugar again after 30 minutes to make sure it has risen. Repeat Step 1 if necessary.

4. Wait 30 to 45 minutes after the blood sugar has returned to normal before driving or operating machinery.

5. Determine how much insulin is still active, using the Unused Insulin Rule in Chapter 17.

Don't Panic and Overeat

Don't go too far. A panic overdose of orange juice with sugar, a box of chocolates or the entire contents of your refrigerator makes your goal of stable blood sugars hard to achieve. These panic attacks come from the release of stress hormones during lows. If your blood sugar frequently goes high after a low, you are eating too much food for your reactions.

Prepare for the panic by having a preset amount of quick carbohydrate from Table 19.3 handy at your bedside, in your pocket or purse, at your desk, in the glove compartment, and handy while exercising. Some people find themselves gaining weight from overtreating reactions, which is another reason to avoid panicking.

A good guide in treating an insulin reaction is to look at how many hours have passed since the last injection of Regular. If the last injection was five to six hours ago, a small amount of carbohydrate should easily correct the low. Here we are assuming the dose of long-acting insulin has been correctly set.

But when an insulin reaction occurs only an hour or two after the last injection of Regular, most of that insulin has yet to act. Therefore more carbohydrate than normal will be needed to treat this low. Of course, if you took 10 units of Regular an hour ago in preparation for a meal and haven't eaten the meal yet, a lot more than 15 or 20 grams of carbohydrate will be needed.

When to reduce your insulin

Consider reducing your insulin doses:

- If reactions are frequent or severe
- If reactions occur within one to three hours after an injection of Regular
- If reactions take more than 15 grams of glucose to bring the blood sugar back to normal
- Before exercise, especially if moderate or strenuous, and it will last longer than 40 minutes
- If you plan to eat a lighter meal than usual
- If you plan to lose weight
- When stress levels drop (as when vacationing)

* If any of these situations arise, call your physician/health care team immediately to discuss lowering your insulin doses.

TO PREVENT INSULIN REACTIONS

Eating Tips

- Eat the meals and snacks that you've taken insulin for.
- Count the carbohydrates in each meal, then match the Carb Regular to these carbohydrates and to the current blood sugar.
- Be careful drinking alcohol. Inebriation and hypoglycemia have a lot in common. Excess alcohol shuts off the glucose normally released from the liver and makes a low blood sugar likely.

Testing Tips

- Test your blood sugar often.
- Learn to use your test results to adjust your insulin doses and carbohydrates. For example, if low blood sugars occur in the afternoon, an afternoon snack, less Regular for lunch, or less long-acting insulin in the morning can help avoid this problem.
- Test often before, during and after exercise. Exercise can lower the blood sugar for as much as 36 hours.
- Always check blood sugars before driving and during long drives.

Be alert for changes in your daily routine (travel, vacation, weight loss, etc.). These can all cause low blood sugars.

Frequent or severe insulin reactions mean that too much insulin is being given. This is especially true if reactions: (1) occur within one to three hours after an injection of Regular, or (2) reactions require more than 15 grams of glucose to bring the blood sugar back to normal. If either of these situations is occurring, call your physician/health care team to discuss an immediate lowering of your insulin doses.

SPECIAL SITUATIONS

Insulin Reactions And Driving

Driving a car can be hypnotic or trancelike. With your attention on the road and other cars, you may not notice that your ability to think, to make decisions, and to interact with others has changed. If your blood sugar has been dropping slowly during a drive, a low blood sugar becomes especially hard to recognize. Don't drive if your blood sugar is below 90 mg/dl (5 mmol) before starting the car, or if it is likely to drop below 90 mg/dl (5 mmol) at any time during the drive.

If you drive a car and become involved in an auto accident due to a low blood sugar, many states will automatically suspend your license!

Always check your blood sugar before driving. Make sure you have glucose tablets, Sweet Tarts,® or other quick carbohydrate easily accessible in your vehicle. Some people always eat some carbohydrate prior to driving just to be safe. On the road, pull over and test your blood sugar if you have any doubts. Don't be a statistic!

Serious Reactions

A serious reaction occurs whenever you are unable to handle the insulin reaction yourself, or you are unable to react appropriately in situations that require your attention, such as driving. Serious situations might involve becoming unconscious or having convulsions. For a severe situation like this, glucagon given by injection is the best treatment. Glucagon is a hormone made by the pancreas, but unlike insulin, glucagon rapidly raises the blood sugar by causing stored glucose to be released from the liver. Commercial preparations of glucagon are a great way to raise low blood sugars.

Glucagon can be used when someone is unconscious or having seizures due to hypoglycemia, when a person is resisting treatment due to hypoglycemia unawareness, when an illness keeps someone from eating, or when nausea prevents eating to correct a low blood sugar.

Glucagon kits are available by prescription and should be kept at home by everyone on insulin. They can be stored at room temperature or in the refrigerator, and are stable for several years after purchase, but dating should be checked periodically to ensure potency.

Someone who is likely to be available during the insulin reaction should be instructed on how to inject glucagon by a Certified Diabetes Educator, a trained nurse, or a pharmacist.

One way to get high blood pressure is to go mountain climbing over molehills.

Earl Wilson

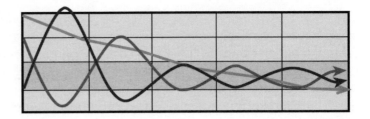

Dangers Of Hypoglycemia Unawareness

20

Research is shedding light on one of the most distressing problems faced by some people who have diabetes (as well as their family, friends and co-workers). The problem, called hypoglycemia unawareness, occurs when a person becomes incapable of dealing with his own low blood sugars. If unnoticed and untreated, hypoglycemia unawareness can create serious problems, including grand mal seizures. If you've ever witnessed seizure activity or bizarre behavior in someone else, you have some idea of the impact this problem creates and its danger.

Hypoglycemia unawareness is not rare. It occurs in 17 percent of those with Type I diabetes. But the risk is far lower in people with Type II diabetes. A study of tight control in Type II diabetes done by the Veterans Administration showed that severe reactions occurred only four percent as often in Type II as compared to Type I.[46]

The lower a person's average blood sugar, the higher their risk for hypoglycemia unawareness. Hypoglycemia unawareness was three times as common in the intensively controlled group in the Diabetes Control and Complications Trial, with 55 percent of these episodes occurring during sleep.

A person with hypoglycemia unawareness loses the ability to think before he notices warning symptoms. By the time the symptoms reach a serious and obvious level, the affected person may still not recognize the obvious shaking, nervousness and sweating. That this could occur during sleep is not surprising, but it also occurs in some people while they are awake.

Normally, the mind recognizes a reaction and allows a person to deal with the dropping blood sugar. However, in certain situations the affected person does not recognize a reaction before it becomes truly severe.

Such situations might be:

- If the blood sugar drop is rapid
- If someone has had diabetes for many years
- If stress or depression are present
- If selfcare is a low priority for any reason

Reaction symptoms become less obvious after having diabetes for several years because the body is less able to release hormones like epinephrine and glucagon. These stress hormones create symptoms like sweating and shaking that make a low blood sugar obvious.

Frequent low blood sugars appear to be the major culprit in hypoglycemia unawareness. One research study showed that stopping frequent lows in people who have hypoglycemia unawareness allowed them to regain awareness of their reactions.[47] Drinking alcohol is also a risk factor for hypoglycemia unawareness. Alcohol contributes to hypoglycemia unawareness in three ways: the mind is less capable of recognizing what's happening, the liver is blocked from creating the glucose needed to raise the blood sugar, and the release of free fatty acids (the backup to glucose for fuel) is also blocked.[48]

The way one loses one's warning signals after a low blood sugar was demonstrated by Dr. Thiemo Veneman and other researchers in an article published in the November, 1993, issue of *Diabetes*.[49] Dr. Veneman and his research group got 10 people who did NOT have diabetes to spend a day at the hospital on two occasions. While they slept, the researchers used insulin to lower their blood sugars to between 40 and 45 mg/dl (2.2 to 2.5 mmol) for two hours in the middle of the night. (No, they didn't wake up! Most of us don't wake up during nighttime reactions. We remember only the reactions we wake up for.) Five people went through a nighttime low on the first visit and the other five on the second visit. In the morning, all were given insulin to lower their blood sugars to see at what point they would recognize symptoms of low blood sugars.

A Few Signs You May Be Having A Reaction...

You are more confused than usual.

You've had your morning coffee.. but you're still cranky and irritable.

You forget simple things... such as your pants.

You're sweaty... but you don't recall working out.

You've got the shakes... and you're not in a draft.

What Dr. Veneman found was that, after sleeping through a reaction at night, people had far more trouble recognizing that their blood sugar was low the following day. Symptoms which warn us that a reaction is occurring come from the release of counter-regulatory hormones. These stress hormones, like epinephrine, norepinephrine and glucagon, were released more slowly and in smaller concentrations following a nighttime reaction (actually after any reaction at all). In other words, a recent low blood sugar depletes us of the hormones that alert us to a reaction and make it more likely that we'll fail to recognize a second low.

Dr. Carmine Fanelli and other researchers in Rome reduced the frequency of insulin reactions in people who had diabetes for seven years or less and who suffered from hypoglycemia unawareness.[51] The subjects raised the target for their premeal blood sugars to 140 mg/dl (7.8 mmol). The frequency of hypoglycemia dropped from once every other day to once every 22 days. The higher premeal blood sugars led to fewer insulin reactions and helped people recognize low blood sugar symptoms.

The counter-regulatory hormone response in these subjects, which alerts them to the presence of a low blood sugar, returned to values that were nearly normal. These researchers demonstrated for the first time that hypoglycemia unawareness is reversible.

Other people can often help someone who suffers from hypoglycemia unawareness avoid a severe reaction by recognizing what is happening and taking appropriate action. If the actions of someone with diabetes on insulin become unusual over a short period of time (usually 10 to 30 minutes), an insulin reaction is the likely cause. Hypoglycemia unawareness may be occurring if the person refuses to acknowledge a problem.

Their actions may be irrational thought, anger, irritability, running away, or insistence that he "feels fine." Thinking is impaired, fight or flight hormone levels are high, and an emotional response is likely. Gentle coaxing and encouragement can often help the person with hypoglycemia unawareness to eat or drink fast-acting carbohydrate. However, confrontation with an individual who already has high stress hormone levels is not wise.

The best way to deal with future episodes of hypoglycemia unawareness is to agree on a plan of action ahead of time. The affected person agrees to test his blood sugar or eat if a supportive coworker or family member gives him a request or special signal. If needed, glucagon can be given by injection by a trained family member, a friend, or even the affected person, to rapidly raise the blood sugar.

Keeping one's blood sugar target slightly higher, avoiding lows, better matching of insulin doses to diet and exercise,

---

How to Prevent Hypoglycemia Unawareness:

- Test blood sugars more often
- Match your insulin doses to your lifestyle
- Set target blood sugars slightly higher
- Be especially careful of a new low during the first couple of days following a reaction

---

and being especially careful following a first reaction are the best ways to prevent hypoglycemia unawareness. Use of the medication acarbose to delay the absorption of carbohydrates has been shown to decrease the risk of insulin reactions. Acarbose, combined with a modest lowering of the Carb Regular is likely to be quite helpful.

For people with an active lifestyle, insulin adjustments may be needed every day to match the variability found in daily life. If insulin reactions occur frequently or if an episode of hypoglycemia unawareness occurs, insulin doses must be lowered immediately. An occasional 2 a.m. blood test can do wonders in preventing hypoglycemia unawareness due to unrecognized nighttime reactions.

If you have ever become unconscious or incoherent due to a low blood sugar and required assistance to treat it, discuss this thoroughly with your physician as soon as possible. You are likely to benefit from working with a physician who specializes in insulin delivery to avoid repeating this dangerous situation.

People tell me one thing and out the other.
I feel as much like I did yesterday as I did today.
I never liked room temperature.
My throat is closer than it seems....
I don't like any of my loved ones.

Daniel M. Wegner's reading test for brain damage

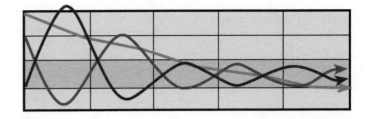

EXERCISE

21

"The only reason I would take up jogging is so I could hear heavy breathing again," says columnist Erma Bombeck. People with diabetes will be happy to know there are even better reasons to exercise.

This chapter explains:

- Benefits of exercise
- Risks of exercise
- How blood sugar and insulin affect exercise
- Effects of different levels of exercise
- Prevention of insulin reactions during exercise

BENEFITS OF EXERCISE

Exercise sharpens the mind and tones the body. It improves heart strength, lung efficiency, endurance, and resistance to stress and fatigue. Exercise helps reduce body fat and improves cholesterol readings. In fact, *not* exercising is considered a major risk factor for heart disease equivalent to smoking a pack of cigarettes a day!

In a study of Harvard alumni, researchers found that the human lifespan increases steadily as exercise levels rise from burning 500 calories a week (couch potato) to 3,500 calories per week (physically fit).[51] The exercise needed to burn 3,500 calories is equivalent to walking three miles an hour for seven hours a week, bicycling 10 miles an hour for five hours a week, or running nine miles an hour for 2.7 hours a week. The more intense the exercise, the less time you need to spend doing it. Benefits are the same.

Moderate levels of exercise when done regularly have been found to protect the heart just as well as strenuous exercise. If you think burning 3,500 calories each week is too much, try participating in moderate exercise regularly. Brisk walking or bicycling for 30 minutes five days a week has been shown to help prevent heart disease.[51] This level of exercise uses 1,000 calories per week and appears to have major benefits for the heart. This is helpful news if you find brisk walking more appealing and safer than running marathons.

AND MORE BENEFITS

Besides its enhancements to lifespan and lifestyle, exercise provides additional benefits in diabetes. Of special interest to those with diabetes are the benefits of exercise to the heart and blood vessels. Because of the higher risk for heart disease with diabetes, the protection offered by exercise is especially important. In addition to this benefit, research conducted at the University of Wisconsin Medical School shows a marked lessening of eye damage in those who exercise.[52] This study ranked groups of people with Type I diabetes according to how much they exercised, then followed them over four years.

When the researchers looked at the amount of eye damage in these different groups, they found that proliferative diabetic retinopathy occurred in 36 percent of women who remained sedentary, but in only 16 percent of those who were very physically active. In men, severe eye damage was 48 percent in sedentary men but only 16 percent in those who were very physically active. Another study also done at the University of Wisconsin found that routine exercise does not worsen existing damage to the retina.[53]

What Is Training?

The American College of Sports Medicine says you are trained when you exercise:

1. Three to five times a week,
2. For 15 to 60 minutes at a time,
3. At 60 to 90% of your maximum heart rate (or 50 to 85% of VO2 max)*,
4. While using any large muscle mass .

* DO NOT USE your heart rate if you have autonomic neuropathy. Discuss this with your physician.

EXERCISE ALSO HAS RISKS

Exercise has very positive benefits, but there are cautions as well. It's smart to discuss any exercise plans with your physician/health care team before starting.

This is especially true if you've had diabetes a long time or have any diabetes-related problems, like nerve damage, eye changes, kidney disease, or a history of heart or blood vessel problems. Blood flow and blood pressure both increase during exercise so that oxygen and fuel can be provided to exercising muscles. Blood flow may increase to 15 or 20 times normal resting levels during strenuous exercise. This could potentially harm organs and blood vessels weakened by past high blood sugars. Risks to blood vessels have to be considered before beginning an exercise program, especially for exercises like weight lifting or diving where the blood pressure is often raised.

If you have nerve damage, you face specific challenges. Nerve damage means pain sensations are not transmitted. The feet can be seriously injured as a result. This does not mean that exercise should be avoided. Rather, you should choose your exercise carefully to protect your feet. Swimming or bike riding would be better in this case than jogging.

Damage to the autonomic nerves that control processes like digestion, heart rate, and blood vessel tone can create an artificially low heart rate and interfere with blood flow to exercising muscles. Autonomic neuropathy also carries with it a higher risk for heart disease. A more gradual training program under supervision is strongly advised when autonomic neuropathy is present.

Hydration is a major concern for any athlete. Water is needed to turn glucose and fat into energy. Dehydration blocks this conversion, and it becomes more likely as blood sugars rise, especially when combined with hot weather. Frequent intake of fluid before, during and after exercise can prevent dehydration.

HOW THE BLOOD SUGAR AFFECTS EXERCISE

Precise blood sugar control during exercise is important not only to health but also to performance. The blood sugar in nondiabetic athletes stays between 70 and 85 mg/dl during even the most strenuous exercise. Reports from athletes with diabetes suggest that their performance is highest when their blood sugars remain close to normal. Normal blood sugars during exercise allow the muscles and heart to receive fuel in the form of glucose and fat in amounts that allow maximum performance. See Table 21.1 for more information.

To improve performance, nondiabetic athletes "fuel up" by eating diets high in carbohydrate. They use carb loading just prior to major exercise events. Diets that are low in

carbohydrate rob the muscles of the glycogen stores they need for endurance and performance. For example, a trained marathon runner on a high carb diet can run for about four hours before exhaustion sets in. But when on a high fat, low carb diet, the same athlete will become exhausted in less than an hour and a half, long before a marathon could be run. Although fat and protein can act as fuels during exercise, endurance begins to suffer if the amounts of fat and protein in the diet are too high.

Athletic performance faces two challenges in diabetes. Performance suffers not only if the diet is low in carbohydrate, but also when the blood sugar goes high or low. To per-

Blood Sugar Level	Effect of Sugar and Insulin Levels on Metabolism	Effect on Performance
less than 65	Too little sugar is in the blood to fuel muscle and brain cells.	Tiredness and poor performance.
65 to 150	Efficient fuel flow.	Maximum Performance
over 150	Sugar has trouble entering muscle cells, especially with low insulin levels.	Performance may be slightly reduced.
over 250	If insulin levels are LOW, blood sugars rise during moderate or strenuous exercise.	Tiredness and poor performance.
over 250	If insulin levels are OK, blood sugars will come down during moderate or strenuous exercise.	Performance varies, exercise may be OK to do.

Table 21.1 Effect of Blood Sugar and Insulin on Metabolism and Performance.

form at his or her best, the athlete with diabetes must accurately judge how to replace the carbs burned and also adjust insulin doses to this activity. Accessing stores of glucose and fat are critical for maximum performance, and insulin controls the availability of these fuels.

Even the amount of oxygen we breath depends on blood sugar control. Research from Austria shows that air flow to the lungs is reduced as much as 15 percent when blood sugars run high.[55] The resulting oxygen deficit would, of course, impair athletic performance as well as be of concern for other health reasons.

How The Body Gets Fuel for Energy

When travelling by car, you can easily determine how much gasoline is needed for a trip. Once you know how long the trip will take (duration), the car's speed (effort or intensity), and the miles per gallon the car gets at that speed, you can calculate the number of gallons of gasoline (energy) needed.

The gallons of gas used in a car trip equal the amount of energy expended during that trip. If you put this same amount of fuel in the gas tank before another similar trip, you won't run out of gas.

Exercise is similar. If someone weighs 150 pounds and runs 30 minutes (duration) at seven miles per hour (intensity or speed), he or she can determine the amount of energy—about 320 calories in this case—used in the run.

The human body is different from a car engine, however, in that it can use two fuels. In humans, either glucose or fat can replace the gasoline used by a car. Over 90 percent of the energy used in exercise comes from these two fuels. The insulin level in the blood is much like a "human carburetor." Insulin adjusts levels of glucose and fat to match the intensity and duration of various forms of exercise. So in essence, both the insulin level and fuel delivery in diabetes must be controlled to keep blood sugars normal.

With diabetes, the simplest way to keep blood sugars normal when exercising is to eat extra carbohydrate. Since carbohydrate is the nutrient most important to performance, some intake of carbohydrate during exercise is usually required. If you know how many carbohydrates are consumed in a particular exercise, you can eat foods containing that number of carbs and maintain control. Insulin doses can be reduced as well to compensate for exercise and *must* be reduced as exercise becomes long and intense.

Exercise Carbs, or ExCarbs, is a system for balancing exercise and is covered in the next chapter. ExCarbs provide a yardstick to measure the impact exercise will have on the blood sugars. ExCarbs are eaten to replace the carbohydrate portion of the fuel burned during physical activity. No insulin is taken to compensate for these ExCarbs. ExCarbs can also be used to guide insulin dose reductions.

How Fuel Works

When starting moderate or strenuous exercise, the first fuel source tapped is the glucose already in the blood, followed rapidly by the glycogen stored in muscle and liver. Glucose is a rapid, easily accessible source of fuel, but the body's supply is limited. During strenuous exercise, the sugar in the bloodstream can be used up in only four minutes compared to 30 minutes at rest.[55] The liver plays the most critical role in supplying glucose for exercise through its release of glycogen as glucose into the bloodstream. These stores, in turn, can be depleted during another 20 to 30 minutes of very strenuous exercise.

The "wall" often encountered by marathon runners at 20 to 24 miles into the race comes from the total depletion of glycogen stores by this demanding exercise. As a way to enlarge these stores, athletes carbohydrate-load before major events by consuming extra amounts of complex carbohydrates. Following these events, glycogen stores are largely depleted and have to be rebuilt. For a 24 to 36 hour period immediately after major events, extra glucose is pulled from the blood to rebuild liver and muscle glycogen stores. This rebuilding is a major reason for the post-exercise hypoglycemia often experienced by people with diabetes.

Body fat acts as the second source of fuel. Fat stores are about 2,000 times as large as the glucose supply in the blood and provide our greatest source of energy. These stores are nearly impossible to deplete.

How Insulin Affects Fuel Delivery

The amount of insulin in the blood helps determine whether carbohydrate or fat will be used as fuel. Too much or too little insulin in the blood causes problems in fuel delivery. For the nondiabetic, these problems are avoided by rapid changes in the blood insulin level. At the start of strenuous exercise, the insulin level drops to half of its pre-exercise level in the first 15 minutes.[56] With moderate exercise, about an hour passes before the same drop in the blood insulin level is seen. This drop in the insulin level allows internal stores of glucose and fat to be released. It also allows the body to switch to fat as the primary fuel, instead of depending on the much smaller supplies of glucose.

Less insulin in the blood:

- Allows the body to burn glucose from glycogen stores in the muscle and liver
- Allows the body to burn some of its fat
- Allows the body to create new glucose

The blood sugar remains steadier when the fuel used in exercise comes from internal glycogen and fat stores. Accessing the fuel in stored fat becomes more important as the length of exercise extends beyond 40 to 60 minutes. Lower insulin levels let fat stores be tapped more easily as energy. They also lessen the chance of a low blood sugar.

By lowering the insulin level, you can exercise longer with less danger of low blood sugars. Because insulin levels are not adjusted automatically for exercise in diabetes, you must set your insulin level carefully to match the level and length of the exercise.

MORE ABOUT INSULIN AND FUEL

We mentioned that the right level of insulin must be maintained to successfully carry out a new exercise program. If insulin levels are too high, sugar enters exercising muscles quickly from the blood, while the release of glycogen from glycogen stores is reduced. The blood sugar drops quickly and an insulin reaction will occur unless the blood sugar was high at the start of exercise or carbs are eaten during the exercise.

On the other hand, if blood insulin levels are too low, stored glucose and free fatty acids are easily released into the blood, but sugar has trouble entering the exercising muscle. This causes the blood sugar to rise during the exercise. Table 21.2 shows some of the effects the insulin level has on blood sugar levels, stress hormone levels, and fuel metabolism.

When the blood sugar is above 250 mg/dl (13.9 mmol), exercise is generally not recommended. This advice is appropriate when a high blood sugar occurs first thing in the morning, as the high blood sugar shows that the insulin level is truly low. Exercising at this time or any time the insulin level is low is likely to raise the blood sugar even higher.

Contrast this to a situation where an athlete prepares for a long athletic event by lowering their Carb Regular and eating extra carbs. Their blood sugar rapidly rises above 250 mg/dl. But in this situation, they can start the event confidently because a quick drop will be seen shortly after they start exercising. They have enough insulin to move the glucose into the exercising muscles.

In this last situation, an alternative to spiking the blood sugar is to reduce both Regular and long-acting insulin sufficiently so that less carbohydrate has to be eaten before the event in order to exercise safely. With a lower insulin level, less carbohydrate is needed at the start of the event. Therefore, the blood sugar does not rise so high. In addition, less eating is needed *during* the event to prevent an insulin reaction because insulin levels have been lowered.

How the Insulin Level Affects Athletic Performance			
Insulin Level:	**Effect on Stress Hormones**	**Effect on Glucose and Free Fatty Acids**	**Effect on Blood Sugar and Performance**
Low	Increased levels of stress hormones	Less glucose enters the muscles. More glucose and free fatty acids are released into the blood. More glucose is produced.	High blood sugar. Poor performance. Possible ketosis.
Ideal	Normal levels of stress hormones	Glucose entry into the muscles is appropriate. Supplies of glucose and free fatty acids are released in the correct amounts.	Normal blood sugar. Optimum performance.
High	Decreased release of stress hormones (until hypoglycemia)	More glucose enters muscle and other cells. Release of glucose and free fatty acids from internal stores is lowered.	Low blood sugar. Poor performance.

Table 21.2 Insulin levels affect performance during exercise

Another example demonstrates the importance of the insulin level. During very strenuous (anaerobic) exercise, like running the 100 yard dash or weight-lifting, glucose provides most of the fuel as it is released very rapidly into the blood, driven by rising stress hormone levels. A similar effect can be seen at the start of competitive aerobic events. This large glucose release from glycogen stores must be rapidly moved into exercising muscle to prevent the blood sugar from rising.

To enable this fast transfer of glucose, the body of a person without diabetes quickly doubles the blood insulin level. But someone with diabetes cannot do this. Instead, he sees a rapid rise in the blood sugar following very strenuous events, even though he starts with a normal blood sugar. Instead of lowering insulin doses as recommended for most exercise, a small dose of Regular may be needed prior to very strenuous exercise to prevent the blood sugar from climbing. Never attempt this without first discussing it with your physician/health care team. You should attempt this particular approach only after extensive testing has demonstrated to you that the extra insulin is really needed.

DIFFERENT LEVELS OF EXERCISE

Mild Exercise

At rest, free fatty acids supply most of our fuel. With mild exercise, like walking or golfing, energy is largely obtained from fats rather than sugar. A drop in the blood sugar is less likely than during more strenuous exercise.

Whether you walk or run a mile makes no difference in the amount of energy used. Moving yourself an identical distance at any speed uses the same number of calories. However, in a one-mile walk, only 20 percent of the calories come from glucose. A satisfying 80 percent of the calories come from fat.

Strenuous Exercise

In contrast to walking, during a strenuous mile run, as much as 80 percent of your calories come from glucose. As few as 20 percent of calories burned come from fat.

As exercise intensity increases, so too does the use of glucose as fuel.

Chromium and Vanadium

The trace minerals chromium and vanadium enhance the glycogen supply in muscle cells, especially when combined with exercise. Chromium helps insulin attach to cell membranes. It reportedly helps in small ways to stabilize blood sugar levels, possibly by enhancing the cell's glycogen buffering system (sort of a shock-absorber for sugars). Exercise also helps to stabilize control by this same mechanism.

In research, vanadium given in large doses has insulin-like effects and reduces the appetite. It rapidly normalizes blood sugars in mice with Type I diabetes. Unfortunately, at the doses required, many of the mice died from the vanadium treatment. Less toxic forms of vanadium, such as one called BMOV, are being tested with some early success.

Short periods of vanadium therapy have been tried in Type II diabetes and found to lower blood sugars and increase insulin sensitvity.[166] Vanadium appears to correct a central defect in Type II diabetes. What doses of vanadium can be used and for how long has not been determined.

Chromium picolinate at levels of 50 to 200 micrograms a day appears to be safe and mildly useful in humans. It has been shown to cause a modest drop in triglyceride levels in people with diabetes.

Because more carbohydrate is used during intense exercise, the blood sugar is more likely to drop. Strenuous exercise, therefore, has to be balanced with more carbohydrate intake or a larger reduction in insulin than mild exercise (except in the case of very strenuous exercise as noted above).

Continuous Exercise

The length of exercise also influences how much carbohydrate is used. Activities that last longer are more likely to drop the blood sugar. For instance, a 30 minute walk might not affect the blood sugar, but walking for 60 minutes may require extra carbohydrate or less Carb Regular.

As exercise continues over time and increases in intensity, the body switches from using its limited stores of glucose and glycogen to using the very large stores of fat as fuel. Figure 21.3

shows this shift in a normal person over several hours. In this example, the person is getting 80 percent of his or her energy from glucose at the start of fairly strenuous exercise. After three hours an equal amount of energy is coming from glucose and fat, but by the end of six hours of exercise these fuels have switched and almost 80 percent of the energy comes from fat.

Remember, though, this person has a *normal* pancreas that automatically lowers insulin levels. If someone with diabetes does not reduce their insulin doses for this same exercise, they will have trouble accessing their body fat as fuel. Instead, they will have to eat carbohydrate to supply this energy.

The numbers on the right of Figure 21.3 show the total amount of energy coming from each source. The total energy used was 3,347 calories, with half of these calories coming from carbohydrate and half from fat. If someone with diabetes kept their insulin level high during this six hour exercise, the excess insulin would blunt their access to internal fat and glycogen stores. With internal stores largely blocked, 3,347 calories coming mostly from carbohydrate would have to be eaten to keep the blood sugar from falling. This is equivalent to eating almost two pounds of pure sugar, or drinking 20 12-ounce cans of regular soda. Obviously, lowering insulin levels helps to prevent both low blood sugars and stomach aches.

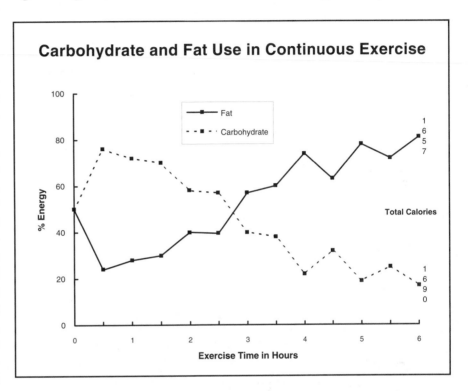

Figure 21.3 The longer the exercise, the more fat is used for fuel

With experience, your ability to estimate how the length and intensity of upcoming activities affect your blood sugar improves, along with your ability to balance them with extra carbohydrate or less insulin.

PREVENTING INSULIN REACTIONS

When low blood sugars occur during and right after exercise or strenuous work, they are usually more difficult to recognize. Symptoms like sweating and shaking can be caused by exercise or by a low blood sugar. Warning signs may go unnoticed because you are focusing on the activity.

To prevent reactions and improve performance, frequent blood sugar monitoring is recommended. Exercise can easily mask the symptoms of a low blood sugar.

More frequent testing can also prevent delayed insulin reactions. These reactions can occur up to 36 hours after strenuous or prolonged exercise or work. They often happen in the middle of the night. Delayed reactions are caused by the gradual drop in blood sugars as the muscle and liver remove sugar to replenish their depleted glycogen stores. To avoid these delayed reactions, test more often, reduce long-acting insulin doses, and eat extra carbohydrate, especially at bedtime.

Keeping high carbohydrate snacks with you during exercise is an important way to prevent insulin reactions. Quick-acting carbohydrate should be handy during any exercise, especially during and after random, intense exercise for which one has not trained. Some examples are canoe trips, backpacking, skiing, horseback riding, spring cleaning, home remodeling, or heavy work in the garden.

Someone who is poorly trained may want to offset exercise with a larger reduction in their insulin doses. This can help the body better access fat for fuel during and after the exercise. Blood sugars should be kept relatively normal, of course. A normal blood sugar during and after the exercise indicates that an ideal balance has been reached between insulin doses and the use of glucose and fat as fuels.

> **REMEMBER:**
> the **LONGER** the exercise,
> the more **INTENSE** the exercise,
> the **LESS TRAINED** you are, and
> the **HIGHER** your insulin level,
> the more likely your blood sugar is to **DROP!**

ADVANTAGE OF PHYSICAL TRAINING

When you do structured exercise on a regular basis, you not only tone up and slim down. Your body uses its fuel more efficiently. The demands on your blood sugar are less when your muscles are well exercised.

When exercising, someone out of shape will use 25 percent more glucose than someone who is in training. The reason is that the fit individual can store a much greater amount of glycogen in his or her muscles. The fit person needs less added carbohydrate in snacks or supplements to prevent insulin reactions.

Of course, the person in good physical condition also benefits by having a healthier body that is less prone to disease. With planning and a little monitoring of the blood sugar, diabetics can approach exercise in a new spirit of fun and enjoyment.

Beginning "New" Exercise

Beginning a new exercise program requires not only that muscle cells rebuild the glycogen used during exercise, but also that they enlarge these glycogen stores to be ready for more of this exercise in the future. This buildup creates larger glycogen stores and makes likely a delayed drop in blood sugar after the exercise, often during sleep that night. Nighttime reactions are more common at the start of any new exercise program or when resuming a previous activity. In time, as training improves and glycogen stores have enlarged, muscle efficiency increases and blood sugars become less likely to drop.

A post-exercise drop is also more likely whenever exercise involves a new muscle group. For example, runners who begin to bike will experience a larger blood sugar drop after biking than after running, even if the energy used for each exercise is the same. This extra drop is caused by the formation of new glycogen stores in the untrained leg muscles that have been used for biking.

Exercise is an important ingredient in anyone's health program, especially someone who also has diabetes. With planning and some blood sugar monitoring, exercise can be experienced with a new spirit of fun and enjoyment.

If at first you don't succeed, find out if the loser gets anything.

Bill Lyon

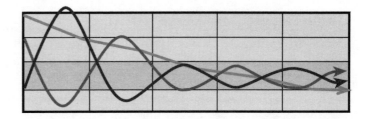

ExCarbs—A New Way To Control During Exercise

22

People with diabetes often associate exercise with loss of control. Like others, they want to exercise because it makes them feel better and improves their health. But what happens? A long walk, some rollerblading or painting the house, and their blood sugar drops. Then a candy bar sends the blood sugar soaring. Some extra insulin to correct the high and the blood sugar goes low again.

Or, perhaps after exercising for a half hour in the morning, the blood sugar rises rather than falls as expected. Or a nighttime low follows a period of exercise during the day.

This chapter will discuss:

- ExCarbs—what are they?

- How to use ExCarbs with exercise

- How to lower insulin doses with ExCarbs

Although absolute rules are not possible with exercise, a concept presented here, called "ExCarbs" or Exercise Carbohydrates, provides a yardstick to measure how a particular exercise affects your blood sugar. ExCarbs provide an easy to understand way to compensate for exercise so you can maintain control. For those who exercise regularly and those who participate in strenuous activity only on occasion, ExCarbs allow control to be maintained with flexible insulin therapy.

The concept is simple. Once you know how many ExCarbs are needed to balance an exercise, you are able to choose among the following:

1. Eating a balancing amount of carbohydrate (easy to do and good for maintaining your current weight)

2. Using ExCarbs to guide the lowering of your insulin doses (great for weight loss)

3. Using a combination of the above (flexible and customized to your needs)

Note that the ExCarbs system is ideally suited to people with Type I diabetes who do not produce any of their own insulin. Instead, they must take all their insulin by multiple injections or via a pump. People with Type II, however, will also find most of this information useful. The amount of carbohydrate used for each type of exercise, listed in Table 22.1, accurately applies to Type II diabetes. However, the 450 Rule used to judge insulin dose reductions will not work for Type IIs because they produce some or all of their own insulin.

Using The ExCarb Table

In Table 22.1, we've translated various exercises into the grams of carbohydrate they are likely to use. This table provides the key information needed to maintain control during various exercises.

Adjustments have been made in the table to compensate for different intensity levels in exercise like bicycling and running. As shown in the last column of the table, fewer calories come from carbs during mild exercise, but as exercise intensity rises so does the percentage of calories that has to come from carbohydrate. Weight is a major determinant of how much energy is used. The table has been set up for weights of 100 lbs., 150 lbs., and 200 lbs. For example, if you weigh 150 pounds and walk three miles in an hour, you'll use 22 grams of carbs. This is equal to an average-sized apple, or to a cup of milk plus a graham cracker.

If you walk at the same pace for two hours rather than one, you'll need 44 grams of carbohydrate. For a 30-minute walk, you will need 11 grams. If, instead of walking, you run the same three miles at a speed of 8 m.p.h., you'll need 53 grams of carbohydrate for a run that lasts only 22 minutes (145 grams times 22 min./60 min.). This is more than twice the amount needed for the leisurely one-hour walk over the same ground!

ExCarbs—Eaten As Carbohydrate

An easy way to keep blood sugars normal while exercising is to eat the amount of carbohydrate that is burned during the exercise. Table 22.1 tells you the number of ExCarbs needed to do this.

Simply look up the exercise you plan and determine how many carbohydrates you need for your exercise. Then eat foods with an equal number of grams of carbohydrate to maintain control. The numbers listed in the table are usually the maximum amount of carbs needed for each hour of exercise to prevent a low blood sugar. Often, less than these amounts are needed right at the time of exercise. But over a 10 to 36 hour period, most or all of these carbohydrates will have to be replaced. (One situation in which these maximum amounts might be needed immediately is when too much insulin is working.)

> **Factors that affect control during exercise:**
> • Recent poor control
> • Length and intensity of the exercise
> • Type of exercise—aerobic/anaerobic
> • Use of abdomen versus muscle areas for injections
> • Training level
> • Timing of exercise relative to meals

This technique of replacing the carbohydrate used as fuel during an exercise requires that you know how to count carbohydrates in food. Counting carbohydrate helps you control your blood sugar more precisely because carbohydrate is the primary component in food that affects the blood sugar. About half of a day's insulin doses are used to balance carbohydrate. If you have forgotten how to count carbohydrates, review Chapter 8.

ExCarbs—Guide To Reducing Insulin Doses

When exercise is short and easy, eating extra carbohydrate is simple and effective. Another way to offset exercise is to lower the insulin doses. As exercise increases in length and intensity, a reduction in the insulin doses becomes more and more necessary. Long, intense periods of exercise require that insulin doses be lowered before the exercise starts, and may require that doses stay lowered for up to 36 hours afterward.

Which insulin to adjust is the next question. Giving less Regular for a meal is ideal for moderate or strenuous exercise that occurs within two hours of eating. When the long-acting insulin is lowered, it takes four to eight hours before the blood insulin actually begins to drop Therefore, these reductions have to be done several hours before an exercise begins.

ExCarbs: Grams of Carbohydrate Used Each Hour in Common Activities

Activity	Grams of carb. used per hour by weight			Approximate % of total calories from Carbs
	100 lb.	**150 lb.**	**200 lb.**	
baseball	25	38	50	40%
basketball				
moderate	35	53	70	50%
vigorous	59	89	118	60%
bicycling				
6 mph	20	27	34	40%
10 mph	35	48	61	50%
14 mph	60	83	105	60%
18 mph	95	130	165	65%
20 mph	122	168	214	70%
dancing				
moderate	17	25	33	40%
vigorous	28	43	57	50%
digging	45	65	83	50%
eating	6	8	10	30%
golfing (pullcart)	23	35	46	40%
handball	59	88	117	60%
jump rope 80/min	73	109	145	65%
mopping	12	18	24	30%
mountain climbing	60	90	120	60%
outside painting	21	31	42	40%
raking leaves	19	28	38	30%
running%				
5 mph	45	68	90	50%
8 mph	96	145	190	65%
10 mph	126	189	252	70%
shovelling	31	45	57	50%
skating				
moderate	25	34	43	40%
vigorous	67	92	117	60%
skiing				
crcntry 5 mph	76	105	133	60%
downhill	52	72	92	50%
water	42	58	74	50%
soccer	45	67	89	50%
swimming				
slow crawl	41	56	71	50%
fast crawl	69	95	121	60%
tennis				
moderate	28	41	55	40%
vigorous	59	88	117	60%
volleyball				
moderate	23	34	45	40%
vigorous	59	88	117	60%
walking				
3 mph	15	22	29	30%
4.5 mph	30	45	59	45%

For example, an exercise that starts mid-morning and lasts for 90 minutes or longer is likely to require less of the breakfast Regular to lower the insulin level during exercise. Likewise, the morning long-acting insulin should be adjusted downward to lower insulin levels following the exercise, during the time that muscle glycogen stores are rebuilt. When exercise is longer and more strenuous, the long-acting insulin may also need to be reduced the night before, especially if UL is used.

Lowering the insulin dose allows more fuel to be obtained from internal stores of glycogen and fat, rather than from eating additional food. This helps those who want to lose weight and those participating in long periods of exercise who don't want to consume the large portions of carbohydrate that would otherwise be required.

Other issues that need to be considered when adjusting insulin doses for the exercise are the current level of training, the duration and intensity of exercise, and the appropriateness of the current insulin doses. Training makes a tremendous difference in the need to adjust insulin. Types of exercise in which you rarely participate are likely to require greater reductions in insulin than those that are routine. People who do regular exercise have already lowered their insulin doses to compensate. Because insulin doses are already lower and glycogen stores have been built up, less adjustment of the insulin dose is needed. But in starting a weekend canoe trip or in starting to train for a marathon, major insulin reductions will likely be needed.

Table 22.1 Use this chart to match your activity with extra carbs

TIMING LOWER INSULIN DOSES

How long before exercise do you need to lower each insulin to ensure that the blood insulin level has been lowered when you start? The type of insulin determines when to lower it. There is always a lag between when an insulin is injected under the skin and when the level of insulin in the blood actually begins to change.

If Regular is lowered for a meal prior to exercise, the blood insulin level begins to "drop" 45 to 60 minutes later. If one wants to lessen the effect from a long-acting insulin, the wait is much longer. These long lag times between when an insulin dose is lowered and when the blood insulin begins to drop will, of course, be shortened when some of the speedier monomeric insulins, like Lispro, become available early in 1996. Table 22.2 provides a timetable to show how long after the lowering of various types of insulin an actual drop in the blood insulin level will begin.

Timing Insulin Reductions

How long before your exercise must you lower each of these insulins to have less insulin in your blood as you begin to exercise?

Lispro	15 to 20 min.
Regular:	30 to 45 min.
NPH or L:	4 to 8 hours
UL:	10 to 24 hours

Table 22.2 When to lower various insulins before exercise

THE 450 RULE AS A GUIDE TO LOWER INSULIN DOSES FOR EXERCISE

ExCarbs can act as a guide to lowering insulin doses. To do this, you need to know how many carbohydrates are equivalent to a unit of Regular. The key to translating carbohydrates into Regular insulin is provided by the 450 Rule for Type I diabetes. This rule says that the number of grams of carbohydrate covered by one unit of Regular can be approximated by dividing 450 by your average total daily insulin dose. (This rule is not an absolute; it provides only an approximation.)

For instance, someone with Type I diabetes who requires 30 total units of insulin each day will need about one unit of Regular for every 15 grams of carbohydrate (450 divided by 30 equals 15). See Figure 22.3. Someone else, who uses 50 units a day, will need about one unit of Regular for each nine grams of carbohydrate (450 divided by 50 equals 9).

Let's try using the 450 Rule to lower Regular insulin doses for exercise. Let's calculate an insulin dose reduction for someone who weighs 150 pounds and uses 38 units of insulin a day. If we divide the daily average insulin dose of 38 units into 450, we get 11.8. If we round this to 12, this person will need one unit of Regular for every 12

The 450 Rule

Use this rule only if you can answer yes to these four questions:

1. Do I have Type I diabetes?
2. Do my long-acting insulin doses make up about half of my total daily insulin dose?
3. Does the other half come from Regular insulin given before each meal?
4. Is my blood sugar control relatively good, i.e., mostly 60 mg/dl to 150 mg/dl before meals? (i.e., is my current insulin dose correct?)

Your Total Daily Insulin Dose	Approximate Number of Grams of Carb Equal to One Unit of Regular:
20 units	22 grams
25 units	18 grams
30 units	15 grams
40 units	11 grams
50 units	9 grams
60 units	8 grams
75 units	6 grams
100 units	5 grams

Table 22.3 Estmates for how many carbs are covered by one unit of Regular

grams of carbohydrate. Here we are assuming they have good control on flexible insulin therapy with physiologic multiple injections, and they take about half of their insulin as NPH, L, or UL.

Now look at Table 22.1. For this person, a 30 minute run at 8 m.p.h. translates into at most 72 grams of ExCarbs (145 grams per hour times a half hour). Knowing this, we can easily figure that the run will be equivalent to 72 grams divided by 12 grams per unit, or a total of six units of Regular.

Our runner can choose to eat extra carbohydrates or lower his or her insulin dose. In the first instance, he eats 72 extra grams of carbohydrate not covered with any additional insulin. These carbohydrates help meet the extra demand for energy the run requires. A good way to replace the ExCarbs is to have about a third of the carbs before the run. The other two-thirds are eaten after the run over several hours. During a longer run, such as a marathon, some carbs would be eaten during the run as well.

In the second instance, our runner reduces his insulin dose. Let's say he or she plans to run an hour after eating. He calculates how many carbs are in his meal and covers his meal with six fewer units of insulin than he ordinarily uses. This way he adjusts his insulin to balance his exercise. Either way will work, but a third way may be better.

Combining ExCarbs and Lower Insulin Doses

A combined approach of eating extra carbohydrates and reducing insulin doses provides the greatest control of blood sugar levels for all but very short periods of exercise.

For example, the 30-minute runner could add 24 grams of extra carbohydrate by eating a banana. He could also reduce his insulin dose by four units, which would take care of the remaining 48 ExCarbs. The runner could even choose to split the insulin reduction between Regular and long-acting. For example, he could lower the breakfast dose by two units of Regular and two units of L or NPH.

Adjustments of insulin and carbohydrate vary greatly from individual to individual. Experimentation, with careful attention to monitoring blood sugars, is the best way to try out these approaches and see which works best for you. Discuss the ExCarb system with your physician before attempting to use it.

How Far Can I Reduce My Insulin Doses?

There are limits to how far insulin doses can be lowered. Let's say your current insulin dose is correct (i.e., your control is quite good). You start a strenuous running program in preparation for a marathon. With multi-mile runs on training days, you find you earn enough ExCarbs to seemingly replace your entire insulin dose. But can your insulin be eliminated if you exercise long enough?

With Type II diabetes, maybe. But with Type I diabetes, definitely not. Let's look at marathon runners who do not have diabetes. During maximum training, their blood insulin level will drop no further than to half of its original level. This tells us that in Type I diabetes, the insulin doses can be reduced no more than 40 percent or 50 percent from the original dose for even the most intense exercise programs.

So keep in mind that, unlike carbohydrates which can be added as needed, insulin doses can be reduced only so far. Even with the most intense forms of exercise, such as running a marathon or competing in a triathelon, the total daily insulin dose cannot be reduced more than 40 to 50 percent. This limit on the lowering of insulin is created by:

1. The need to cover meal carbohydrates with enough insulin to keep the blood sugar from rising after a meal.

2. The need for sufficient background insulin to allow glucose to enter cells, and keep the massive internal stores of glucose and fat from being released.

Of course, never take any dose of insulin that seems inappropriate. If you usually take three units of Regular for your meal prior to the start of your exercise and your blood sugar control has been great, never take more or less than this amount, even if suggested by the ExCarb system, the 450 Rule, or any other rule. Your blood sugars are always your best guide.

WHEN TO USE EXCARBS

The ExCarb table shows how many total carbs are required, but we also need to know *when* to replace them. Even if the blood sugar is normal before exercise, all of the carbohydrates needed are not eaten immediately. For example, during the first 30 minutes of moderately strenuous exercise, like running at 6 m.p.h., half of the fuel comes from carbs. But during this run, about 40 percent of this 50 percent comes directly from internal glycogen stores in the leg muscles. The remaining 10 percent comes out of the blood as glucose. Only the glucose obtained from the blood has to be *immediately* replaced through eating, or from the production and release of glucose by the liver. Even when insulin levels are high during a 30 minute run, only 16 percent of the calories come directly from the blood as glucose.

During the first 30 minutes of exercise, local muscle glycogen contributes about five times as much glucose as the blood does. As the run continues beyond 30 minutes, more and more glucose begins to be pulled directly from the blood. The amount of glucose coming directly from the blood climbs gradually during the first couple of hours to about 40 percent. This is why eating or drinking carbohydrate becomes more important as exercise continues and why the blood sugar is more likely to drop.

Diabetes Athletes Association

The International Diabetic Athletes Association (IDAA) holds a terrific three-day North American Conference each year with talks and workshops by diabetes specialists involved in a wide variety of sports.

One finding presented by several exercise specialists and confirmed by participants, is that the more muscle mass one has, the easier blood sugar control becomes.

This suggests that a combination of aerobic exercise for cardiovascular fitness and strength training for muscle mass is important in diabetes.

IDAA: 1647-B West Bethany Home Road; Phoenix, Arizona 85015; (602) 433-2113; (800) 898-4311.

The insulin level drops about 50 percent for the nondiabetic during the first two hours of moderate exercise. In diabetes, if insulin levels do not drop, more food is required to keep the blood sugar from falling. Eating becomes the major way to supply fuel when insulin levels are set too high.

Most of the carbohydrate burned when exercise lasts less than 30 to 45 minutes comes from nearby internal stores rather than the blood. If insulin levels are correctly lowered when an exercise starts, these internal glycogen stores can begin to release their stored glucose as fuel for the exercise. After the exercise, the glycogen stores are rebuilt over a 3 to 36 hour period through a gradual removal of sugar from the bloodstream.

The longer and more intense an exercise, the longer it takes to rebuild muscle glycogen stores afterwards. The blood sugar may drop for periods as long as 36 hours after the exercise. This means that not all of the carbohydrate used in exercise have to be eaten immediately. Most athletes with diabetes add carbs to their bedtime snack to prevent a nighttime drop.

COMBINED ADJUSTMENTS

Eating ExCarbs and lowering insulin doses are two ways to balance exercise. What about combining them? General recommendations for combined carbohydrate and insulin adjustments are given in Table 22.4. Both the intensity and duration of exercise affect how it can be balanced with ExCarbs or reduced insulin doses. Basically, the longer and the more strenuous an exercise, the greater the adjustment required, and the more likely that insulin doses will have to be lowered.

The length of exercise is easy to determine, but intensity is a different matter. Intensity is highly specific to each individual. Two people may be running side by side at the same speed, but one may be running at maximum intensity, while for the other the same exercise may be mild.

"Mild" exercise is any extra activity that is relatively easy for you to do, such as casual walking. "Moderate" exercise involves something that makes you breathe harder, but which you could do for some time, such as brisk walking or jogging. "Intense" exercise involves anything that causes deep breathing, but still allows you to carry on a conversation. Examples are race walking or a steady, fast bike ride. Table 22.4 gives recommendations for adjusting carbohydrates, Regular insulin, and long-acting insulin to match exercise of different duration and intensity.

Adjustments of insulin and carbohydrate vary greatly from individual to individual. The reasons for these variations from one person to the next are complex and not completely understood. Some people may lower their doses of Regular and long-acting insulin only slightly for exercise; others may find that a large insulin reduction is the only way to control their blood sugars. For some, the breakfast Regular does

---

Fast versus Slow Carbs

Not all carbs are the same. Different foods raise the blood sugar at different speeds. These speed differences can be useful.

Fast carbs are ideal for raising low blood sugars before or during exercise, and also for balancing exercise that uses carbs rapidly.

Slow carbs help prevent drops during longer periods of activity. They can be eaten before an exercise starts and every 45 minutes thereafter. Here are some examples of each:

Faster Carbs: Glucose tablets, Sweet Tarts, honey, corn flakes, raisin bran, athletic drinks (Exceed, Body Fuel), raisins, dried or ripe fruits, regular soft drinks, apple juice.

Slower Carbs: Athletic bars (PowerBar, PurePower), oatmeal, Swiss muesli, Cheerios, fruit, Fig Newtons, Teddy Grahams, ginger snaps, pasta al dente, brown rice, candy bars (high in fat).

---

not need to be lowered for morning exercise, but when they do the same exercise later in the day, they have to reduce their insulin. The only way to determine your own response is to experiment, record your results, and discuss these with your physician/health care team.

Once you have determined the ExCarbs (Exercise Carbohydrates) needed for your exercise, you can offset this need by:

- Eating that number of grams of carbohydrate
- Reducing the Meal Regular
- Reducing the long-acting insulin
- Allowing the exercise to lower a high blood sugar
- Some combination of the above

Let's say you weigh 200 pounds, use 45 units of insulin a day and generally have good control. From Table 13.1 in Chapter 13, you'll need one unit of Regular for each 10 grams of carbohydrate and one Regular for each 33 points you wish to lower your blood sugar. You wake up one morning with a blood sugar of 166 and want to eat 100 grams of carbohydrate for breakfast, then ride a bike at 14 m.p.h. for one hour. If you weren't riding, you would take 10 units for your breakfast, plus another two units for the high blood sugar.

From Table 22.1 you calculate that at 200 pounds and riding 14 m.p.h. for an hour, you'll need the equivalent of 105 grams of ExCarbs for the ride. These 105 grams can be translated into these choices:

- An extra 105 grams of free carbohydrate during the day
- 10 fewer units of insulin (105grams/10 grams per unit)
- A blood sugar drop of 333 points (33 point drop per unit X 10 units)
- Some combination of the above

Two good choices:

1. Take your normal dose of insulin—10 units for breakfast, plus the two extra units for the high blood sugar. Then eat 100 grams of carbohydrate for breakfast, plus another 105 grams of free carbohydrate during and after the bike ride. (The extra carbohydrate equals *seven* average slices of bread.)

2. Or take five units of insulin to cover breakfast (50 percent of the usual breakfast Regular) and 1 unit to lower the blood sugar. Then eat your usual 100 grams of carbohydrate for breakfast. (Less insulin allows better access to internal glycogen stores). Only 50 grams of carbohydrate will then be needed during and after the ride.

THE TALK TEST

One measure of exercise is the "talk test". As long as you can talk during your exercise, it is an aerobic exercise. If you cannot carry on a conversation while exercising, your effort is beyond intense and into the anaerobic ("without oxygen") range. Examples of anaerobic exercise are the 100-yard dash and power weight lifting. During short periods of anaerobic exercise, the blood sugar can rise despite seemingly adequate insulin levels because glucose is mobilized very rapidly from glycogen stores to supply fuel. This can overwhelm the current insulin level and cause the blood sugar to go up. If experience shows that the blood sugar rises after this type of exercise, check with your physician for more specific instructions on insulin adjustments.

Carb and Insulin Adjustments (for 100 lb. athlete)									
Exercise Duration	Exercise Intensity								
	Mild			Moderate			Intense		
	ExCarbs	Regular	L/N/UL	ExCarbs	Regular	L/N/UL	ExCarbs	Regular	L/N/UL
15 min.	No Adj.	No Adj.	No Adj.	No Adj.	No Adj.	No Adj.	20 gm*	20% less	No Adj.
30 min.	No Adj.	No Adj.	No Adj.	30 gm*	No Adj.	No Adj.	40 gm*	30% less	No Adj.
45 min	20 gm*	No Adj.	No Adj.	35 gm*	30% less	No Adj.	50 gm*	50% less	No Adj.
60 min	25 gm*	30% less	No Adj.	40 gm*	30% less	No Adj.	60 gm*	50% less	20% less
120 min	50 gm*	30% less	No Adj.	70 gm*	50% less	20% less	110 gm*	70% less	40% less
240 min	80 gm*	30% less	20% less	120 gm*	70% less	20% less	200 gm*	70% less	40% less

* Important Note on ExCarbs: You MUST ADJUST THESE FIGURES to your own weight! At 200 lbs, you'll need TWICE as many ExCarbs. Remember to test these values to determine your actual need.

Table 22.4 Estimates for carb and insulin adjustments to balance exercise

WRONG INSULIN DOSES

What if the ExCarb system doesn't work? Don't feel bad! There are lots of competing factors that can influence the blood sugar during exercise. A key question to ask if the ExCarb system is not working is, "Are my current insulin doses set properly?"

An example of someone with insulin doses set too high is a person who has frequent low blood sugars in the afternoon, but who decides to start exercising at 3 p.m. anyway without first lowering their insulin dose or eating extra ExCarbs. The insulin reaction that follows will now be quite severe, but should not be blamed on the exercise. Blame it instead on the underlying excess insulin.

Another example of excess insulin would be someone who takes a large dose of Regular just before eating a meal with lots of carbohydrate. Even though this dose of Regular matches the carbs in the meal, two hours later the blood sugar has risen to 300 mg/dl (16.7 mmol) because the injection was taken just before eating. The person, confident he is safe because of the high reading, goes out for a six mile run. The severe insulin reaction 45 minutes later should not be blamed on the exercise but on too much insulin.

An example of insulin doses set too low is someone who wakes up in the morning with a reading of 180 mg/dl (10 mmol), and then goes jogging for 30 minutes. She is surprised when her blood sugar rises to 240 mg/dl (13.3 mmol) on her return. Again, the exercise is not to blame. Rather, the underlying lack of insulin allows the glycogen stores in the liver and muscle to break down rapidly. But because the insulin is low, glucose has trouble moving into the muscles for use as fuel. Her blood sugar control might have been improved by taking a small dose of Regular before starting to jog, or, even better, by maintaining blood sugar control during the previous night.

STRESS HORMONES

Another less predicable factor is the effect of stress hormones. Large amounts of stress hormones are often released at the start of a competitive event, like a swim meet, a 10K run, or a century bike ride. Nervousness or jitteryness at the starting line is a sign of stress hormones at work. Blood sugars can often rise unexpectedly in these circumstances.

UNUSUAL CIRCUMSTANCES

Problems can also creep in when exercise conditions change. If you usually walk two miles on flat ground, but decide to walk the same distance in hilly country, you'll use more fuel in climbing these grades. A strong headwind can increase carbohydrate consumption by about one percent for each extra mile per hour of headwind (i.e., for a 10 m.p.h. headwind, increase carbs by 10 percent). Walking in dry sand or soft snow can easily double the amount of carbohydrate needed for the same walk on firm ground.

Activities that have uneven pacing, like spring-cleaning or football, can also cause problems. It's hard to predict whether you'll spend the next hour sorting through the closet for throwaways or moving furniture. Or if you'll spend the entire game on the bench or on the field. Luckily, most activities don't suffer from this unpredictability.

EXERCISE WISELY

Keep in mind your previous experiences with similar exercise. Make sure your insulin doses and carbohydrate intake are matched to your normal daily lifestyle, before attempting to make further adjustments for exercise.

Discuss your exercise program with your physician/health care team, monitor your blood sugars often, and use all the information and tips on exercise provided in this book.

Test your blood sugar more often when exercising. This feedback lets you adjust your insulin doses more precisely to the length and intensity of your exercise. For rapid correction of low blood sugars during exercise, carry some fast-acting carbohydrates, like glucose tablets or SweetTarts.®

If you plan to participate in a strenuous activity like a triathelon, marathon, century, etc., tap the experience of other athletes with diabetes who have encountered these challenges before you. You can usually get a quick referral to another athlete who participates in your sport through the International Diabetic Athletes Association at (602) 433-2113. Discuss your findings with your physician.

Exercise can make you feel and look younger, especially if you learn how to master your blood sugar control in the process. Exercise also appears to be an important way to reduce the risk for complications and to live a long, healthy life.

For Control During Exercise, Think:

1. How long and hard am I going to exercise?

2. How many ExCarbs will I use? (see Table 22.1)

3. What's my current insulin level? Frequent highs, lows, or both?

4. Do I want to use my ExCarbs as food to eat, as a guide to reduce my insulin doses (Table 22.3)*, or as a combination of the two (Table 22.4)*?

Never adjust insulin doses on your own without discussing these changes with your physician.

More Exercise Tips For Serious Athletes

- Test blood sugars more often while exercising and in the following 24 to 36 hours.

- Lower insulin doses before long periods of exercise or work for better access to internal stores of glucose and fat. (This also helps prevent low blood sugars.)

- For performance and safety, keep the blood sugar between 70 and 150 mg/dl (3.9 to 8.3 mmol) during exercise and try to keep it from dropping below 65 mg/dl afterward.

- The longer and more strenuous an exercise, the more likely the blood sugar will go low, and the greater the need to lower insulin doses.

- The less trained one is, the more likely the blood sugar will go low.

- *Very strenuous* and anaerobic exercises may raise the blood sugar if glucose is mobilized faster than it can be moved into cells by the prevailing insulin level.

- For exercise that lasts less than an hour and occurs within three hours of a meal, you can:
    1. Eat extra ExCarbs, or
    2. Lower the normal Carb Regular by 30 percent to 50 percent, or
    3. Reduce the Carb Regular by 20 percent and eat fewer ExCarbs.

- Normal doses of Carb Regular may need to be lowered by 50 percent or more when taken before or during vigorous exercise or heavy work. For example, if one unit is normally taken for each 10 grams of carbohydrate, try taking only one unit for every 18 or 20 grams when working or exercising hard. Some vigorous exercise may require the total elimination of Regular for the carbohydrate in a meal.

- Regular taken to bring down high blood sugars may also need to be lowered by 40 percent to 70 percent when given before or during periods of moderate or strenuous exercise.

- For intense activities that last a day or two, such as a weekend backpacking trip, try lowering the long-acting insulin dose by 20 percent to 40 percent and the Carb Regular by 50 percent. Lower the long-acting insulin eight to 12 hours ahead of the activity for Lente or NPH, and 20 hours for Ultralente. Keep it lowered for about 24 hours following the exercise.

- The long-acting insulin dose rarely needs to be lowered for short, random periods of exercise, but may need to be gradually reduced as physical fitness increases.

- Remember, never lower your total daily insulin dose more than 50 percent for even the most strenuous exercise.

- **Be sure to discuss these suggestions with your physician before making any changes in your own insulin doses. These suggestions may not be appropriate for you.**

An excellent diet cannot make an average athlete great,
but a poor diet can make a great athlete average.

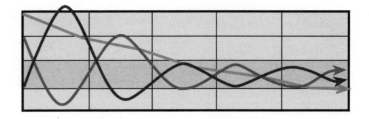

PREGNANCY AND DIABETES

23

Some three to four percent of all pregnancies are complicated by gestational diabetes—that is, diabetes which begins during the course of a pregnancy. It appears late in the second trimester or in the third trimester. In the United States, 90,000 women face this health challenge every year. Another 10,000 births occur in women who have Type I diabetes prior to conceiving. These 100,000 women are highly motivated to control their diabetes to promote the health and well-being of the child (and, ultimately, their own health).

In this chapter, we'll present an approach which uses flexible insulin therapy to stabilize blood sugar control and reduce the swings in blood sugars that can occur from diet and use of insulin. We'll cover:

- Complications related to diabetes and pregnancy
- The importance of blood sugar control to a healthy outcome
- How to prepare for pregnancy with existing diabetes
- Gestational diabetes
- How insulin requirements change
- Better control with the Rule of 18ths

PREGNANCY COMPLICATIONS

For good health a person with diabetes needs to keep blood sugar levels normal or close to normal all the time. This is not the time to be on a rollercoaster. During pregnancy, control becomes more important because only strictly controlled glucose levels can create the environment needed to produce a healthy baby. High blood sugar levels during the first eight weeks of pregnancy are associated with serious birth defects. High levels in the second and third trimesters may result in fetal complications and problems at birth.

First Trimester Complications Include:

- Birth defects
- Spontaneous abortions

The risk for these complications increases when diabetes is already present but poorly controlled before conception (either Type I or Type II diabetes).

Second and Third Trimester Complications include

- Premature delivery
- Delayed growth and development
- Large birth weight (more than 9 pounds) requiring a Cesarean section
- Severe low blood sugars in the infant after delivery
- Respiratory distress syndrome
- Enlarged heart
- Low calcium level and tetany (jitters)
- Jaundice
- High red blood cell count

These complications may occur with poor control in any type of diabetes.

More Information On Complications

One negative outcome of high blood sugars is that the baby does not have fully developed lungs even if he/she is large at birth. This causes the child to have respiratory distress or difficulty in breathing after delivery.

Another unwanted outcome is severe low blood sugars in a baby. This happens when the fetus produces large amounts of insulin to compensate for the mother's high blood sugars. When the baby is born and separated from the mother's high blood sugars, he/she continues to produce excess insulin for several days, causing the severe low blood sugars.

Blood Sugar Goals During Pregnancy

Before meals and at bedtime:	60-90 mg/dl (3.3-5 mmol)
1 hour after atarting to eat:	120 mg/dl (6.7 mmol)
2 a.m.-6 a.m.:	60-90 mg/dl (3.3-5 mmol)

Note: Keep your HbA_{1c} at least 20% below the laboratory's upper limit for normal for non-pregnant women (i.e., in the normal range *for pregnancy*)

Table 23.1 Target Blood Sugars Before And During Preg-

The risk for all of these complications is greatly reduced by a mother who maintains normal blood sugars throughout the pregnancy. Women with Type I or Type II diabetes who plan to conceive should keep their blood sugars at the same levels recommended for pregnancy.

Control Problems in Pregnancy

Control of the blood sugars is made more difficult during pregnancy for several reasons: First, the blood sugar of a nondiabetic, pregnant woman is normally lower than a woman who is not pregnant. Therefore the proper target blood sugars for the pregnant woman with diabetes are also lower and closer to the hypoglycemic range. The HbA_{1c} levels should be maintained within the normal range for pregnancy (i.e., a range that is 20 percent lower than the "normal" normal—each lab's normal range will vary). Furthermore, problems such as nausea and vomiting caused by morning sickness, and the increasing demands for insulin as weight rises also make blood sugar control more difficult.

Blood sugar control has been directly linked to the survival of the infant since 1949. Priscilla White, M.D., reported from the Joslin Clinic in Boston that 18 percent of the children of mothers with diabetes were stillborn or died shortly after birth. However, she noted that "good treatment of diabetes" clearly improved the outcome.[57] By 1965, Jorgen Pedersen, M.D., studied pregnant women in Copenhagen. Those women who had none of the "Bad signs" in Table 23.2 had a 6.9 percent rate of fetal and neonatal deaths.[58, 59] In contrast, in 130 diabetic pregnancies where one of these signs was present, the death rate rose to 31 percent.[60]

Things To Avoid In Pregnancy
1. Hospitalization for ketoacidosis,
2. Pre-eclampsia (also called toxemia of pregnancy: a combination of high blood pressure, headaches, protein in the urine, and swelling of the legs, usually late in the pregnancy),
3. Kidney infection, or
4. Neglect of prenatal care.

Table 23.2 Dr. Pedersen's "Bad Signs"

During the late 1960s and early 1970s it became clear that the higher the average glucose level of the mother, the higher the risk that the child would be lost near birth.

By the 1980s, it was possible to normalize the mother's blood sugars and the child's metabolic environment through blood sugar testing at home. However, in women with Type I diabetes, birth defects emerged as a major cause of infant deaths.[61, 62] In various studies, birth defects were found to occur in four to 11 percent of infants born to women with Type I diabetes, compared to a rate of 1.2 to 2.1 percent in the general population.[62, 63, 64] Researchers and physicians realized that the blood sugar in these women had to be normalized *before conception* because the child's organs were formed within the first 8 weeks after conception.

Several researchers also noticed that higher HbA_{1c} values during the first trimester were associated with more spontaneous abortions than were seen in normal women.[65, 66] Interestingly, one researcher found that women who have excellent control throughout pregnancy actually have a lower rate of spontaneous abortions.[66] An HbA_{1c} that is normal or no higher than one percent above the upper limit of the normal range will minimize the risk of birth defects and spontaneous abortions.

In Type I diabetes, if the demands for insulin are not met, the greatest threat to the fetus and the mother are high blood sugars leading to ketoacidosis. If the mother develops severe ketoacidosis, there is a high probability—up to 95 percent—that the fetus will die. Obviously, frequent blood sugar monitoring and working closely with specialists in diabetes and pregnancy are keys to success.

What if my blood sugar is high before a meal?
Take the Carb Regular plus enough High Blood Sugar Regular to lower the high reading. Check the blood sugar every 30 minutes until it is below 120 mg/dl (6.7 mmol) before eating. If the blood sugar is still high two hours later, take additional High Blood Sugar Regular. If you cannot delay eating, eat the fat and protein portions first, and have the carbohydrate as late into the meal as possible to allow the reading to drop.

PREPARING FOR PREGNANCY

A woman with Type I diabetes should have blood sugar levels under control before she plans to conceive. Once the HbA_{1c} is in the normal range, the uterus is ready to receive an embryo! Every effort is made to keep the blood sugar normal throughout her pregnancy. (See Table 23.1 for targets.) The ideal pregnancy management program includes the following:

- Frequent blood glucose and HbA_{1c} tests to determine the exact level of control
- An eye exam for retinopathy
- A 24-hour urine collection for creatinine clearance, total protein and microalbumin to assess the health of the kidneys, done each trimester
- An evaluation of her cardiovascular system
- A detailed diet program, using the Rule of 18ths (see Table 23.4).
- A regular exercise program.

Although existing damage to the eyes, kidneys, or vascular system does not rule out a healthy pregnancy, it does carry a greater risk of complications for the mother and the child.[67]

Until the blood sugars are ideal to ensure the best possible outcome, adequate birth control must be prescribed. Low dose birth control pills appear to be both safe and effective.

The reason that the prospective Type I mother should achieve excellent control before conception is that, as soon as the egg is fertilized, the cells start dividing. The fetus begins to develop specialized organs and tissues. This occurs within the first three months of pregnancy and determines more than anything else whether the baby will develop normally. High blood sugars interfere with cell division and can lead to DNA damage.

All women planning a pregnancy can benefit from eating healthy, exercising regularly, and supplementing the diet with a vitamin/mineral capsule designed for pregnancy.

GESTATIONAL DIABETES

The most common form of diabetes during pregnancy, gestational diabetes, develops during an otherwise normal pregnancy due to the stresses that pregnancy places on the body. Gestational diabetes usually appears in the second trimester, because the second trimester is the time in which the stresses of pregnancy begin to place demands on insulin production. So critical is it to catch any elevated blood sugar that the current recommendation is that all pregnant women be screened with a shortened glucose tolerance test. This is routinely done in pregnant women between the 24th and 28th weeks (the sixth month) of pregnancy.

High risk individuals for gestational diabetes include women who are overweight, have a history of multiple stillbirths and miscarriages, have previously delivered babies weighing more than 9 pounds at birth, or have a strong family history of diabetes.

These women should have a glucose tolerance test done as soon as

Can Insulin Harm The Child?

Some women are concerned that injected insulin will harm the fetus. This cannot happen because the majority of the insulin does not pass through the placenta, and what does pass is not biologically active. However *glucose* passes easily through the placenta. As the child's own pancreas develops and begins producing insulin during the second and third trimester, he/she will try to lower the high blood sugar he/she is exposed to by producing its own insulin. Because insulin is a growth hormone, these excess amounts cause the child to grow and add unneeded weight. Macrosomia (or "large body") develops and can make delivery difficult or dangerous for both mother and child.

the pregnancy is discovered, and repeated at 24 to 28 weeks gestation if the first test was negative. These tests are done to detect any high blood sugars: a fasting serum glucose above 105 mg/dl (5.8 mmol) or a blood sugar above 140 mg/dl (7.8 mmol) at two hours after a meal. This testing is necessary because there is a 20 percent chance that the infant will die or develop complications if control is achieved only by the second trimester.[68] Testing is done before conception and throughout the pregnancy if the woman is high risk and attempting to conceive.

After the birth of the child, the metabolism of someone with gestational diabetes often returns to normal, or to an "impaired glucose tolerance" treated with diet and exercise. There is a 50 percent chance that someone who's had gestational diabetes will develop diabetes within the next 20 years. Those who had a prediabetic condition, called impaired glucose tolerance, before pregnancy will likely have it afterwards.

INSULIN REQUIREMENTS DURING PREGNANCY

When the woman with well-controlled Type I diabetes becomes pregnant, she will adjust her normal insulin dose. If she has Type II diabetes, she may inject insulin or control her diabetes with diet. When a Type II becomes pregnant, if she is on a diabetes pill, the medication is immediately replaced with insulin, since oral agents may have a negative effect on the fetus. (In fact, if the pregnancy is planned, she should switch from a pill to insulin before conception.) The blood sugars of the person with diet controlled diabetes should be monitored carefully at home and in the clinic according to Table 23.1. Insulin will almost certainly be needed at some point in the pregnancy. Insulin is started whenever the blood sugar rises above the targets.

Typical Changes in Insulin Doses by Trimester*				
If your weight is:	**Pre**	**1st**	**2nd**	**3rd**
100 lbs.	27	32	36	41
120	33	38	44	49
130	35	41	47	53
140	38	45	51	57
160	44	51	58	65
180	49	57	65	74
200	55	64	73	82

* Insulin requirments in many women with Type II diabetes or gestational diabetes often start at these doses, then quickly increase due to the needs of the woman.

Table 23.3 Insulin requirements for Type I diabetes through pregnancy

Insulin requirements rise steadily over the course of the pregnancy, and usually double during the pregnancy.[68] This rise is caused by several factors—weight gain, increased caloric intake, creation of new tissue, and an increase in hormones that conflict with the actions of insulin. Each woman's experience varies. A very strict regimen of blood glucose monitoring done at least 8 times a day must be maintained to quickly alert the woman and her health care team to an increased need for insulin. These checks should occur before each meal, an hour after beginning each meal, at bedtime and at 3 a.m. Table 23.3 shows the rise in insulin requirements throughout the pregnancy for a woman with Type I diabetes.

The one exception to this general rise in the need for insulin occurs during the last four weeks of pregnancy. Then, insulin needs may drop! During the last month, the fetus starts drawing out more glucose from the mother's blood for its needs. A larger bedtime snack is often required to keep the blood sugar from dropping during the night. The daytime Regular may have to be reduced also if the mother is unable to eat a substantial meal because of the enlarging uterus. However, if your need for insulin suddenly drops, not caused by these obvious reasons, this can be an ominous sign. *Contact your obstetrician for consideration of immediate delivery.*

Flexible insulin therapy, with combined long-acting and short-acting insulins, works best for maintaining control in the face of a constant rise in the need for insulin, especially in the last 4 months of pregnancy. The usual dose is an injection of Regular and Lente or NPH in the morning before breakfast, Regular before lunch, and an injection of Regular and Lente or NPH before dinner, or Regular before dinner and the Lente or NPH at bedtime.

Additional Regular should be used anytime necessary to bring down a high blood sugar quickly so the fetus is not harmed. Increased doses are usually required every 5 to 15 days as determined by charting the blood sugars and the amounts of carbohydrate eaten. A graphical charting system, like Smart Charts, is highly recommended during pregnancy to track everything that may be affecting control.

A woman with gestational diabetes will need to start insulin as soon as her blood sugars rise above the range in Table 23.1. Insulin doses for gestational diabetes must be handled on an individual basis. Some women are more sensitive to insulin, many are more resistant. A starting point is to use total insulin doses similar to those found in Table 23.3. Insulin demand and blood sugar patterns in gestational diabetes vary a great deal and have to be matched to each person's need.

NAUSEA AND INSULIN

Nausea and vomiting often occur in the first trimester. The pregnant woman with Type I diabetes may think that if she does not eat, she doesn't need any insulin. This is not the case. The liver continues making glucose even when someone doesn't eat. Insulin is needed to keep the blood sugar from rising even if no food is eaten.

With flexible insulin therapy, the Lente or NPH insulin works to keep blood sugars normal while a person is not eating. This long-acting insulin should be taken, even if nausea prevents eating.

Glucagon should be kept available for use anytime the Carb Regular has been taken for a meal that the woman is unable to eat due to nausea. Glucagon raises the blood sugar by causing the liver to release some of its stored glucose. Of course, when nausea is frequent, the woman may want to take only part of the premeal Regular, and then attempt to eat 30 minutes later. If food can be eaten at that time, the rest of the injection can be taken. If food or caloric drinks cannot be kept down, a partial dose of glucagon can be injected at that time to raise the blood sugar.

Glucagon: How Much Do You Need?
Each 0.15 mg of glucagon (or 1/6 of the standard 1 mg. dose) raises the blood sugar 30 mg/dl!

CARBOHYDRATE ADJUSTMENTS DURING PREGNANCY

Eating a balanced diet is more important for a pregnant woman with diabetes than it is for a nondiabetic pregnant woman. Because the fetus is continually removing glucose from the mother's blood for growth, eating many meals and snacks throughout the day is also important.

During pregnancy, a diet comprised of 40 percent carbohydrate, 40 percent fat, and 20 percent protein is generally recommended. The carbohydrate portion is spread throughout the day to make blood sugar control easier. An easy way to spread these carbohydrates is by using the "Rule of 18ths." A woman, with the help of her dietician, estimates her total daily caloric need. The carbohydrate portion is then distributed throughout the day (see Table 23.4).

As an example, someone who requires 1800 calories per day will eat 180 grams of carbohydrate. This total of 180 grams divided by 18 (Rule of 18ths) equals 10 grams per 18th. According to the table, her breakfast would be 20 grams of carbohydrate.

The breakfast carbohydrate is kept low in comparison to the rest of the day. Most people with diabetes have a Dawn Phenomenon to some extent, and because of this are more resistant to insulin at the beginning of the day. Keeping food intake low until noon time helps in dealing with this. Since strict control is of such importance, staying away from high glycemic foods which can spike the blood sugar is a good idea.

A woman's caloric need rises throughout the pregnancy, usually adding between 500 and 1,000 extra calories per day. These calories supply fuel for her higher metabolic rate and her required weight gain. The distribution of carbohydrates changes along with the calorie change. Table 23.5 provides guidance for distributing the carb portion of these calories.

Carb Distribution With The Rule of 18ths		
Meal or Snack	**Portion of The Day's Total Carbohydrate:**	**Percent of Total Daily Carbs**
Breakfast	2/18	10%
Midmorning Snack	1/18	5%
Lunch	5/18	30%
Midafternoon Snack	2/18	10%
Dinner	5/18	30%
After Dinner Snack	2/18	10%
Bedtime Snack	1/18	5%

Table 23.4 How carbs are disbursed with 18ths

How To Distribute Carbs As Calorie Need Rises In Pregnancy

		Total Calories							
	18ths	**1600**	**1800**	**2000**	**2200**	**2400**	**2600**	**2800**	**3000**
40% as Carbs (grams)		160	180	200	220	240	260	280	300
Breakfast	2/18	18	20	22	24	26	29	30	34
Midmorning Snack	1/18	9	10	12	14	14	14	16	17
Lunch	5/18	44	50	55	60	66	72	78`	82
Midafternoon Snack	2/18	18	20	22	24	27	30	31	34
Dinner	5/18	44	50	55	60	66	72	78	82
After Dinner Snack	2/18	18	20	22	24	27	29	31	34
Bedtime	1/18	9	10	12	14	14	14	16	17

Table 23.5 Grams of Carbohydrate in Each Meal as Calories Rise During Pregnancy

Labor And Delivery

During active labor at the hospital, muscle contractions can be similar to strenuous exercise and reduce insulin need dramatically. The goal is to maintain blood glucose levels between 60 and 100 mg/dl. To attain this, the long acting insulin may need to be quickly reduced and the Regular is often discontinued. An intravenous line is started with insulin added as needed to lower the blood sugar and glucose added to raise it. Hourly blood sugars are done to determine if the insulin or the glucose needs adjusting.

After Delivery

When the baby has been delivered, the hormones in the placenta that antagonize insulin are removed. Insulin requirements rapidly drop and insulin is usually no longer required in someone with gestational diabetes. The reduced demand for insulin after delivery, together with the prolonged "exercise" of labor may be so dramatic that even in Type I diabetes insulin may not be needed for a day or two. In a few days, the woman with Type I diabetes will be back to normal insulin requirements, approximately the same as before the pregnancy.

Breast Feeding And Type I

If the mother breastfeeds (highly recommended for its benefits to the baby's immune system), insulin requirements may be lower than before conception because more glucose is needed for breast milk. The mother has to adjust her own calorie intake to match the child's breastfeeding habits. If the baby consumes most of its calories at bedtime or in the middle of the night, the mother must do the same. Many women need only a few units of longer-acting insulin in the evening with this breastfeeding pattern.

A Personal Note:

In my own experience over the last 15 years, I have seen more than 500 babies born to mothers with diabetes in one or another of the intensive care programs that I have been involved with. The mothers followed the recommendations in this chapter. None of the babies had any of the problems typical to infants of mothers with diabetes. Luckily, remembering these children's names has become easy, because half of the babies are named Lois!

Lois Jovanovic-Peterson, M.D.

BLOOD SUGAR PATTERNS AND SOLUTIONS

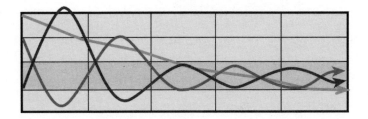

BLOOD SUGAR PATTERNS
RECOGNIZING AND CORRECTING CONTROL PROBLEMS

24

Remember the Smart Charts in Chapter 6? By recording your blood sugar levels daily, you begin to see a pattern. With flexible insulin therapy, you are able to correct the problems these patterns reveal.

This chapter will show you:

- Typical problem patterns
- How to correct these problem patterns

Identifying patterns in your blood sugars is a critical step for control. These patterns can occur every day, several days in a row, or they may occur only occasionally. Suggestions for solving them are given below each pattern. For repeating patterns (i.e., high all the time or often low in the afternoon), insulin dose adjustments are usually needed. If the pattern is occasional, the solution is a one-time fix that can be reused in the future when needed. Blood sugars to the left of the charts are shown in both mg/dl (U.S.) and mmol (Canada, Europe, and others) values.

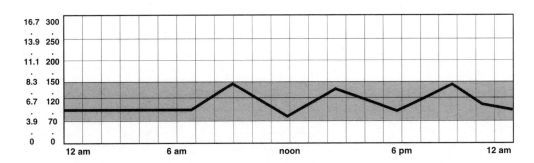

PATTERN: NORMAL

WHAT TO DO: Nothing, keep up the great work!

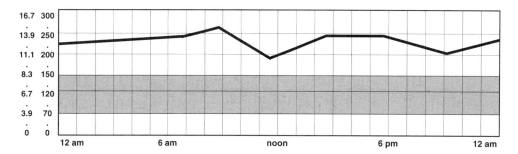

PATTERN: HIGH

WHAT TO DO: Raise insulin. Review diet, exercise and weight for improvements. Consider infection, pain, stress, bad insulin, steroid or new medication.

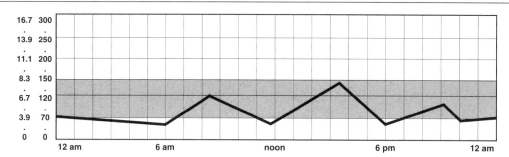

PATTERN: LOW

WHAT TO DO: Lower the insulin doses; eat more carbohydrate.

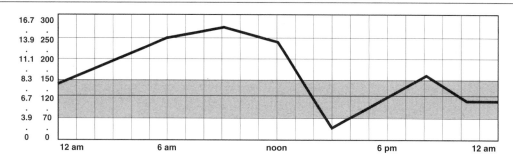

PATTERN: HIGH TO LOW—overcorrecting highs with too much Regular

WHAT TO DO: Less High Blood Sugar Regular; review the Unused Insulin Rule; test more often and eat before the blood sugar drops.

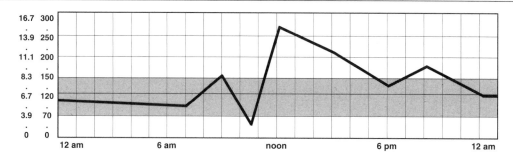

PATTERN: LOW TO HIGH—overcorrecting low blood sugars by overeating

WHAT TO DO: Use glucose or Sweet Tarts® and eat less for lows. Remember: one gram of glucose raises the blood sugar 3 to 5 points.

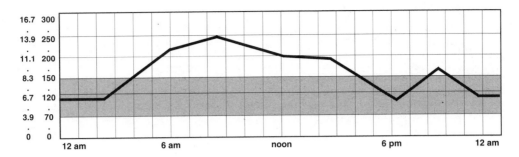

PATTERN: DAWN PHENOMENON

WHAT TO DO: Increase bedtime dose of long-acting insulin

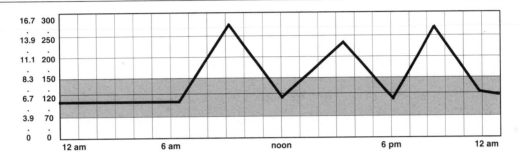

PATTERN: SPIKES BETWEEN MEALS

WHAT TO DO: Take Carb Regular earlier; raise long-acting insulin slightly; split daily Carbs into snacks and meals; eat lower glycemic index foods; add high-fiber items (psyllium, guar gum) to meals.

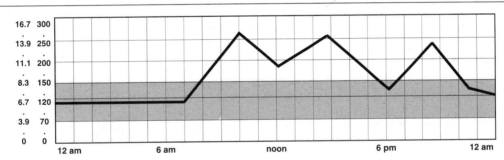

PATTERN: HIGH AFTER MEALS

WHAT TO DO: Raise Carb Regular; eat less carbohydrate; exercise after the meal; take Carb Regular at least 30 minutes before eating.

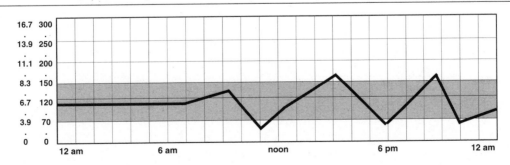

PATTERN: LOW AFTER MEALS

WHAT TO DO: Lower Carb Regular; increase carbohydrates.

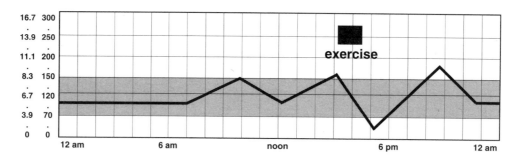

PATTERN: EXERCISE LOWS

WHAT TO DO: Lower the insulin and/or increase carbohydrates with exercise.

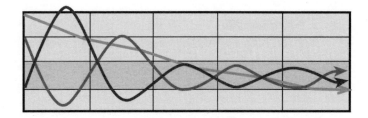

How To Correct Highs Before Breakfast

25

The first blood sugar of the day is the most important one for determining the entire day's control, but it's often the hardest to bring into the normal range. This is especially true if you have a Dawn Phenomenon or have Type II diabetes. Waking up with a high blood sugar after going to bed with a normal reading can be very discouraging. Flexible insulin therapy can help you recognize abnormal overnight blood sugar patterns, and help you adjust your insulin to correct them.

In this chapter, we'll explore:

• Causes for waking highs

• How to correct them

High Blood Sugars Before Breakfast

Why does a high morning blood sugar throw off the rest of the day? Largely because it results from a low insulin level in the blood. This signals the liver to produce excess sugar! In the nondiabetic, a low insulin level accompanies a low blood sugar. When the liver senses a low insulin level, it responds by releasing sugar into the blood. In diabetes, the liver responds the same way to the low blood insulin level even though the blood sugar is already high! Once this process starts, it becomes difficult to stop and causes extra sugar to be produced and released through the morning hours.

If you take extra insulin for a high morning blood sugar, be careful of afternoon lows. When two or more doses of High Blood Sugar Regular accumulate during the morning and early afternoon, an insulin reaction later in the day becomes likely. Then gorging on food in the panic of the insulin reaction can cause the blood sugar to rise again and repeat the cycle. *And you're on the rollercoaster!*

Five common causes for high blood sugars before breakfast with corrections are presented.

Too Little Overnight Long-Acting Insulin

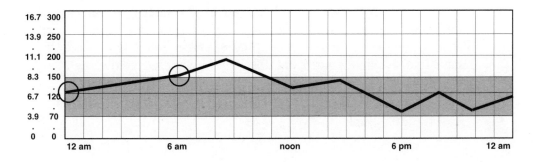

A blood sugar rises during the night because the overnight long-acting insulin dose is too low. Too little background insulin is present to keep the blood sugar controlled.

Test: At these times. If you frequently get the following results, your high morning blood sugar is caused by too little nighttime long-acting insulin.

Bedtime: Normal blood sugar.

2 a.m.: Usually midway between the bedtime and waking blood sugars.

Waking: Always higher than the 2 a.m. and bedtime readings.

Action: Raise the evening dose of long-acting insulin to provide more overnight coverage. You may wish to review Chapter 14 and you can test a new dose as described in Table 14.1. Be cautious when raising your nighttime insulin. If you've had nighttime reactions in the past, discuss this carefully with your physician (A bedtime dose is safer.). As you adjust, test the blood sugars more often, especially at 2 a.m. Also be careful of afternoon lows when correcting the higher morning readings with extra Regular.

A HIGH PROTEIN DINNER

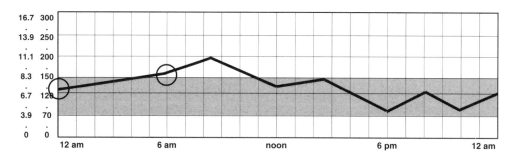

This pattern is similar to the previous one, but its cause and its treatment are different. When protein is eaten, 40 to 50 percent of it will change slowly into glucose over a period of several hours following the meal. The protein in most meals has little influence on blood sugar levels. When *large amounts* of protein are eaten, however, this often causes the blood sugar to rise overnight. Examples of heavy protein intake would be an 8 to 12 ounce steak, a Mexican dinner with a lot of refried beans, or an evening snack of several ounces of nuts.

Test: At these times. If you typically get the following results after a high protein meal or snack, the protein is causing your high morning blood sugars.

Bedtime: Normal blood sugar

2 a.m.: Usually midway between the bedtime and waking blood sugars.

Waking: Always higher than the 2 a.m. and bedtime readings.

Action: 1. Limit the protein in evening meals.

2. Consider taking slightly more long-acting insulin on evenings that you eat high protein meals to offset the increased production of glucose from the protein. Then cover any high bedtime readings with High Blood Sugar Regular (use half of your usual dose if you want to avoid a nighttime reaction).

3. If necessary, wake up halfway through the night, check your blood sugar and correct it if it is high.

If you must eat a high protein meal and you can predict that this meal will raise the blood sugar overnight, then adjust your evening insulin doses. If you can't predict the meal's effect, you may want to wake in the middle of the night and correct the blood sugar then, if necessary. If your experience is limited, testing at 2 a.m. is the best way to avoid a nighttime insulin reaction.

A High Bedtime Blood Sugar

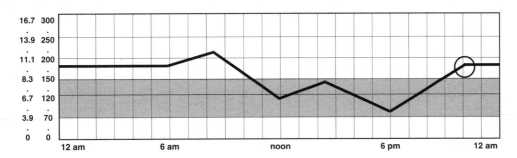

This pattern is easy to identify because the blood sugar is high in the morning only because it was already high the night before at bedtime.

Test: At these times. The following results point to a high bedtime blood sugar as the cause of the high morning reading.

Bedtime: High

2 a.m.:   High

Waking: High

Action: First, be sure the overnight long-acting insulin has been tested and correctly set. Be sure to fully cover the carbohydrate eaten during the evening hours. If the blood sugar is high at bedtime, take sufficient Regular to help bring it down, but not enough to cause a nighttime reaction. For bedtime injections, be sure to use the Unused Insulin Rule in Chapter 17 to estimate how much Regular insulin is still working from the dinner injection. Test the blood sugar at 1 a.m. or 2 a.m. to prevent a nighttime low blood sugar. If you are keeping your bedtime reading high because you are concerned about having a reaction during the night, discuss this situation with your physician/health care team.

The Dawn Phenomenon

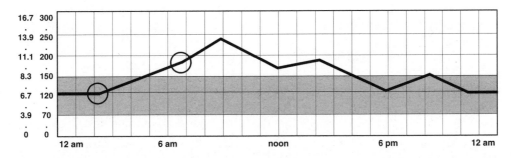

The Dawn Phenomenon pattern shows the need for extra long-acting insulin in the early morning hours. Ideally, the blood insulin level would rise between the hours of 1 a.m. and 3 a.m. to prevent this early morning rise (for those who sleep typical nighttime hours).

Test: At these times. The following results point to a high morning blood sugar caused by a Dawn Phenomenon.

Bedtime: Normal blood sugar.

2 a.m.: Close to the bedtime blood sugar, lower than the waking reading.

Waking: Much higher than the 2 a.m. and bedtime readings.

Action: Increase the long-acting NPH or Lente taken at bedtime or dinner. (UL is not used with the Dawn Phenomenon because it has little peak.) The best effect is seen when you raise the blood insulin level one to two hours before the blood sugar usually starts its own rise. Although it is not a true Dawn Phenomenon in Type II diabetes, a high morning reading is often a problem. A trick those with Type II diabetes can try is to eat a long-acting carbohydrate, like a green apple or raw cornstarch, at bedtime. This will often help lower a slightly elevated morning reading. In Type II, a long-acting insulin, given before dinner (usually with Regular) or at bedtime, is often needed.

More Information on this Pattern

Among people with Type I diabetes, 50 percent to 70 percent need some extra insulin beginning between 1 a.m. and 3 a.m. to control a Dawn Phenomenon. About 20 to 30 percent need substantially more insulin to keep the breakfast reading controlled. Be sure to check with your physician/health care team to make sure you have a Dawn Phenomenon before increasing your long-acting insulin taken in the evening.

High morning blood sugars are very common in Type II diabetes, although the reason for the high readings is somewhat different. People with impaired sensitivity to insulin, as often happens with Type II, tend to release more fat into the blood during the night when eating has stopped. Fat makes cells less sensitive to insulin. The liver begins to think that insulin levels have dropped. Because a low insulin level is interpreted as a low blood sugar by the liver, it starts to make glucose to raise the blood sugar! Due to these crossed signals, the liver makes unneeded glucose, causing the person to wake up with a high blood sugar.

OVERTREATING A NIGHTTIME INSULIN REACTION

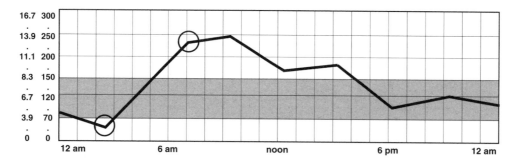

It's hard to be rational after waking in the middle of the night from stress hormones released during an insulin reaction, especially when brain cells aren't getting enough fuel to think clearly. In the fear and confusion that follows, emptying the refrigerator may seem normal and reassuring. Overeating in the wee hours, however, results in sky-high blood sugars the following morning, and often for several hours into the day.

Test: At these times. Thes following results suggest that your high morning blood sugar is caused by overtreating a nighttime insulin reaction.

Bedtime: Varies; can be low, normal or high.

2 a.m.: Low to very low, followed by excessive eating (over 25 to 30 grams of carbs)

Waking: Always high after eating too much for the low.

Action: The best solution is to determine why the nighttime reactions are occurring and prevent them. Lower the evening long-acting insulin, the dinner Regular, or High Blood Sugar Regular given in the evening if one of these doses is the culprit. The second best solution is to keep glucose or quick-acting carbohydrate beside the bed and use it routinely to treat all nighttime reactions. Even in the middle of the night, it is hard to overdose on glucose tablets.

Frequently (half the time in most research studies) people do not wake up during a nighttime reaction. If someone sleeps through a reaction in the middle of the night, the morning blood sugar will rarely rise any higher than 150 mg/dl, *unless* the dose of long-acting insulin for the early morning hours is too low. If you have high blood sugars in the morning, and are blaming them on reactions during the night, test your blood sugar a few times at 2 a.m. to find out. Also see Chapter 19 for the signs that this may be occurring.

SAMPLE LONG-ACTING INSULIN DOSES

Two examples for doses of the long-acting insulin are shown in the figures that follow. These doses depict ways in which background insulin, given as two injections of a long-acting insulin, might be needed by two different people during a 24-hour period when little or no food is eaten.

Both people need 20 units of long-acting insulin during a day. These examples are only models for background insulin doses. The way in which your own long-acting insulin doses are given is likely to be quite different.

To Balance A Steady Need For Insulin

A constant background insulin level is a good place to start for many people. This satisfies insulin need in 30 to 40 percent of the population, and will closely approximate need in perhaps another 20 or 30 percent.

Figure 25.1 shows a constant background need for insulin: a straight, level line indicating the need for insulin at a constant level through the entire day. This need can usually be best provided with two injections of Lente or Ultralente which have a flatter peak in their activity than NPH. (In the example that follows, the person uses 10 units of UL before breakfast and dinner to cover their background insulin need.) NPH can also be considered to match this steady background need, but because NPH has a more distinct and earlier peak in its activity, it will not give as flat an insulin level (Of course, its activity can be spread more evenly through the day by taking three injections of NPH, rather than two). Injections are ideally timed so that any peaking of the insulin occurs at meal times.

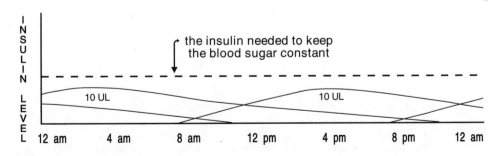

Figure 25.1 Doses To Match A Constant Background Need For Insulin

To Offset A Dawn Phenomenon

Figure 25.2 shows sample long-acting insulin doses to match insulin need in someone with a Dawn Phenomenon. Between 50 percent and 70 percent of people with diabetes need additional insulin in the blood during the early morning hours to offset a Dawn Phenomenon. This increasing demand for insulin during the night, usually noticed as a rise in the blood sugar between 3 a.m. to 9 a.m., is caused by an increased release of growth hormone.[69] People with a Dawn Phenomenon often need to have extra long-acting insulin in the blood beginning at 2 a.m. to 3 a.m.

To prevent the Dawn Phenomenon from raising the blood sugar, long-acting insulin is injected at bedtime or at dinner to get the blood insulin level starting to rise before the blood sugar begins its own rise. Control can be improved when the insulin level is raised before the liver begins to produce excess glucose at around 3 a.m. There is, however, some additional risk of nighttime lows when insulin levels are raised too early during the night.

Before attempting to cover a Dawn Phenomenon, discuss proposed changes in the nighttime long-acting insulin carefully with your physician/health care team. Extra caution is required when raising nighttime insulin doses due to the risk of nighttime lows. *Never assume you have a Dawn Phenomenon without first discussing this with your physician.*

In the example, this individual used 12 units of NPH at bedtime to cover the Dawn Phenomenon with another 8 units of NPH before breakfast.

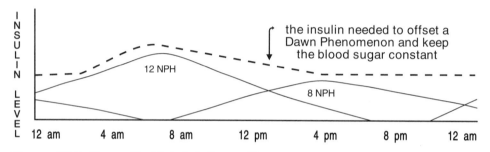

Figure 25.2 Doses To Match A Dawn Phenomenon

You may find that you have a Dawn Phenomenon with occasional nighttime reactions. You can diagnose this problem by testing at 2 a.m. This situation requires decreasing the long-acting insulin working in the first part of the night to prevent the insulin reactions, but increasing it in the early morning to stop a blood sugar rise from the Dawn Phenomenon. Always stop the nighttime lows first. The safest way to treat this is to inject the long-acting insulin at bedtime or in some cases to switch from NPH to Lente (with its slightly later peaking) at dinner. Some reduction in the Carb Regular for dinner may also help you avoid middle of the night lows.

Insulin doses that match a constant need for long-acting insulin or the Dawn Phenomenon will work for most people. But if blood sugars are not controlled with either of these approaches, many other approaches are available, depending on the time of the day that blood sugars are poorly controlled.

When everyone is out to get you, paranoia is only good thinking.

Johnny Fever
WKRP Cincinnati

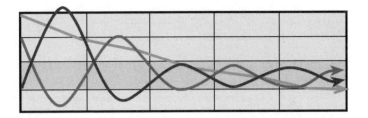

How To Correct Highs After Meals

26

In the previous chapter, we looked at the causes of and remedies for high blood sugars before breakfast. In this chapter, we'll look at people who have a normal blood sugar before a meal, but then lose control when it rises sharply after eating.

This chapter covers:

- Causes for high blood sugars after eating
- How to correct these highs
- Unrecognized nighttime reactions as a cause for post-breakfast highs

Except for the last example that is specific to breakfast, these remedies can be applied to any meal of the day where blood sugar control is poor.

Inadequate Or Missed Carb Regular

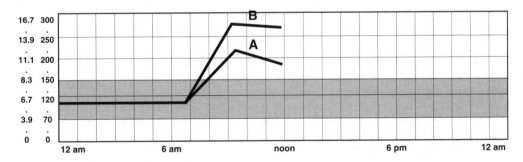

Here the Carb Regular taken before a meal was too little for the carbohydrate eaten (line A), or was missed entirely (line B).

What Happens: You can frequently underestimate the ratio of insulin to carbohydrate if you don't count your carbs. Less frequently, you might misjudge the dose of insulin to take for a meal, such as in a restaurant. In most cases, too little insulin is being taken for the food. Forgetting to take a dose of insulin is—hopefully—infrequent.

Action: Retest your ratio of grams of carbohydrate to each unit of Regular to be sure that you are getting the right amount of Carb Regular for your meals. Also review Chapter 8 on carb counting to be sure you have a good understanding of this excellent tool. At many restaurants, nutritional information is available to guide your doses. A little attention to meals that consistently give you problems will lead to a solution.

CARB REGULAR TAKEN JUST BEFORE EATING

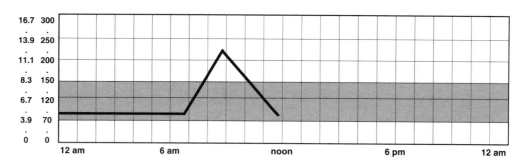

What happens: Regular insulin takes at least 20 to 30 minutes to have any effect, and at least 2 1/2 to 3 hours before it peaks in its activity. In contrast, carbohydrate creates an almost immediate rise in the blood sugar. When Regular is taken just before a meal, the carbohydrate raises the blood sugar before the Regular has a chance to counteract it and a high blood sugar follows. This high blood sugar then returns to normal before the next meal, as the insulin finally has its desired effect.

This pattern is common when injections are taken just before meals. How high the blood sugar goes depends on the person's sensitivity to insulin, the amount of carbohydrate eaten, how active they are after the meal, and the glycemic index of the foods eaten.

Action: Try using the faster Lispro insulin when it becomes available. With Regular, take the injection 30 to 45 minutes before eating. If unable to take Regular early, try one or more of the following: subtract carbohydrate from the meal and add it as a snack, add fiber like psyllium or guar gum to the meal to slow down the digestion of carbohydrates, or get extra exercise just after eating. Another option is to use the medication acarbose (Precose) before the meal to slow down the digestion of carbohydrate.

A FAST-ACTING CARBOHYDRATE IN THE MEAL

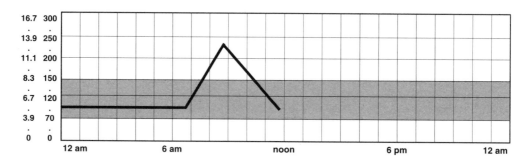

What happens: This pattern is similar to the last one. But instead of an injection that's taken too late, here a fast-acting carbohydrate causes the blood sugar to spike before the Carb Regular taken for the meal can enter the blood. Many foods have a high glycemic index. That is, they raise the blood sugar quickly after meals, even though no more carbohydrate than usual is eaten.

If you eat 70 grams of carbohydrate for breakfast as old-fashioned oatmeal, your blood sugar isn't likely to rise dramatically. If you eat a typical cold cereal, it probably will. Many typical breakfast foods, like cold cereal with a ripe banana, instant oatmeal, yogurt with a fruit syrup, or a toasted cheese sandwich, will spike the mid-morning reading.

Action: Check the glycemic index of the suspected food in Appendix B. Partially or totally replace the fast-acting carb with slower ones—those that have a low glycemic index—such as old-fashioned oatmeal, high fiber cereals, strawberries, or plain yogurt with fresh fruit sliced into it.

Other possible solutions:

- Try using the faster Lispro insulin.
- Take the Carb Regular *more than* 30 minutes before meals that contain fast carbs
- Eat less carbohydrate for the meal; then add a carbohydrate snack a couple of hours later
- Add fiber like psyllium or guar gum before the meal
- Get extra exercise after the meal.
- Use the medication acarbose (Precose) before the meal to slow down the digestion of carbohydrate.

All of these problems, too little Carb Regular, an injection taken too close to the meal, and fast carb foods can occur at any meal of the day. The solutions can also be applied to any meal of the day. The next situation is more specific to the breakfast meal.

AN UNRECOGNIZED NIGHTTIME REACTION

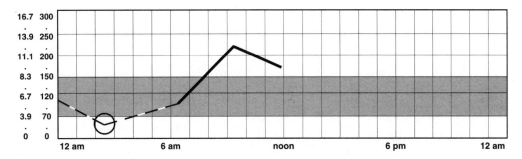

What happens: This pattern is typical for the morning hours following an unrecognized nighttime reaction due to a significant release of stress hormones during the reaction. Notice in this pattern that the blood sugar may often be normal before breakfast. Review Chapter 19 for signs of nighttime reactions.

This pattern occurs even when someone correctly covers the breakfast carbohydrate with Regular. The usually adequate dose of Carb Regular is blunted by the stress hormones released during the nighttime reaction, and the blood sugar rises. Stress hormones can raise blood sugar levels for eight to 10 hours after a major reaction. The blood sugar may remain high at lunch and into the afternoon.

Action: Learn to recognize the symptoms of nighttime reactions. Determine the cause of the reaction and correct the evening insulins if necessary. Check your blood sugar at 2 a.m. if you're not sure of the cause. As an ounce of prevention, it's smart to do a 2 a.m. or 3 a.m. test every two weeks even when you're not having any problems.

Never argue with people who buy ink by the gallon.

Tommy Lasorda

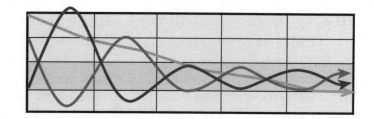

How To Correct Afternoon And Nighttime Lows

27

If you have low blood sugars at night or in the late afternoon (the most common times for lows), this chapter should provide helpful solutions.

How To Prevent Nighttime Lows

The lowest blood sugar of the day in people taking insulin is most likely to occur around 2 a.m. In one study of people on both conventional injections and multiple daily injections, researchers found that people with diabetes had a low blood sugar every fourth night on average.[70] Nighttime lows are more common in Type I diabetes, but they also occur in those with Type II diabetes, especially in Type IIs where sensitivity to insulin is higher.

One reason for nighttime reactions is that people are most sensitive to insulin between midnight and 3 a.m. The liver seems to play a major role both in this decreased need for insulin in the middle of the night and also in the increased need later before dawn. The liver lowers its glucose production in the middle of the night and then begins to increase it 2 to 4 hours before waking. Another reason for nighttime lows is the accumulation of insulin from the daytime hours, especially from the dinner Regular, the evening long-acting insulin, and even the morning long-acting insulin.

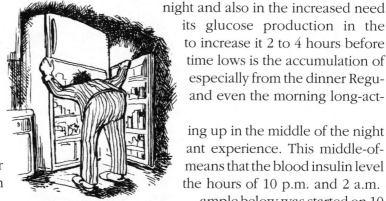

Although he was usually a sound sleeper, frequent nighttime lows had forced Lewis into a familiar nocturnal position.

Regardless of the cause, waking up in the middle of the night shaking and sweating is not a pleasant experience. This middle-of-the-night drop in the blood sugar means that the blood insulin level needs to be lowered, usually between the hours of 10 p.m. and 2 a.m.

The individual in the example below was started on 10 units of Lente before breakfast and dinner, but changed the doses after discussing it with his/her physician. The dose of Lente at dinner was dropped to 7 units with a balancing rise to 13 units in the morning Lente dose. (A second option this person can try is to move the injection of Lente from dinner to bedtime.)

	Breakfast	Lunch	Dinner	Bed
Nighttime lows	6R/10L	6R	6R/10L	
First option	6R/13L	5R	7R/7L	
Second option	6R/13L	5R	7R	7L

How To Avoid Nighttime Lows With A Dawn Phenomenon

Some people require less insulin in the middle of the night to avoid lows, but also need more insulin before waking to prevent their blood sugar from rising due to a Dawn Phenomenon. This is more likely in Type I and in Type II sensitive diabetes. The blood insulin level often has to be reduced at 9 or 10 p.m., then raised higher than the daytime level at 1 a.m. to 3 a.m. At 9 to 11 a.m., the background insulin level is lowered back to normal. If this blood sugar pattern is present, the doses of either the dinner Regular or dinner long-acting insulin must be reduced to avoid nighttime reactions (the first option below), or the evening insulin must be given at bedtime to better match the morning blood sugar rises (second option). Insulin doses to match this need are shown below:

	Breakfast	Lunch	Dinner	Bed
Nighttime lows and Dawn Phenom.	6R/10N	6R	6R/10N	
First option	6R/10L	6R	5R/9L	
Second option	6R/10N	6R	6R	10N

How To Avoid Afternoon Lows

Another common problem is someone who needs less insulin in the afternoon to prevent low blood sugars. These individuals are often physically active or are taking their largest dose of long-acting insulin in the evening to control a Dawn Phenomenon. These afternoon lows often occur when an excess of insulin has built up in the blood from injections given the evening before and from Carb Regular given for breakfast and lunch. This can happen in Type I or Type II diabetes.

To avoid these lows, less long-acting insulin is given in the morning so that the blood insulin level will be reduced during the afternoon (first option below). Another way to accomplish the same thing is to give less Regular than usual for the carbohydrate eaten at lunch (second option). Someone might reduce their insulin to solve this problem as follows:

	Breakfast	Lunch	Dinner	Bed
Afternoon lows	6R/10N	6R	6R	10N
First option	6R/8N	6R	6R	10N
Second option	6R/10N	4R	6R	10N

With the more precise insulin delivery found with flexible insulin therapy, it becomes easier to adjust long-acting insulins to meet these differing demands. Some people, particularly those who exercise strenuously or for prolonged periods, benefit from frequent insulin dose adjustments to match changes in their activity level. More activity, less insulin; less activity, more insulin. Almost everyone requires some periodic adjustments in their insulin doses, including the long-acting insulin. Changes in activity level, season and weight in particular create the need to change doses.

With experience, you will be making these changes as needed. Be sure to consult with your physician/health care team if you are uncertain what your own blood sugar results mean.

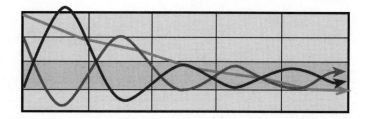

TROUBLESHOOTING VARIABLE BLOOD SUGARS

28

When blood sugars are often high at a certain time of day, such as at bedtime, this is an abnormal pattern, with a cause that is usually easy to track down. We showed you how to find such causes in the previous chapters.

Truly variable blood sugars, on the other hand, have little identifiable pattern to them and can happen even when using flexible insulin therapy. Though flexible insulin therapy provides the best opportunity for stable blood sugars, it does not guarantee this. A variable blood sugar is one that frequently strays outside the 70 to 140 mg/dl (3.9 to 7.8 mmol) range before meals and beyond 200 mg/dl (11 mmol) after meals. In addition the blood sugar readings show little pattern at the same time of day.

This chapter deals with some of the causes for variable blood sugars, including:

- Insulin reactions
- A variable lifestyle
- Problems with carbohydrates
- Stress

SEEK THE SOURCE

If you've caught the rollercoaster and are feeling very frustrated with your lack of control, it is important to remember that there is always a source for this variability. First calm down and put on your thinking cap. Then ask yourself the questions in Figure 28.1. Be quite honest with your answers.

If you answered "yes" to several items or quite emphatically to one of them, you can improve your control by dealing with the areas of your life marked with "yes." As you regulate habits, prevent lows and lessen stress, your charts will take on a pattern. A recognizable pattern can be analyzed for solutions.

INSULIN REACTIONS

In some people, frequent insulin reactions are causing their variable blood sugars. When too much insulin is being given and insulin reactions are overtreated by panic eating, variable blood sugars are the result. The extra insulin used to treat the highs caused by panic eating can lead to even more insulin reactions.

Insulin re-actions are easy to recognize as the source for variable blood sugars on your charts. A pattern of frequent low blood sugars is typically followed by unusually high readings one to four hours later. If these highs of-ten go above 150 mg/dl, panic eat-ing may be the reason. If the

Finding the Cause of Variable Readings

If your control is poor and you see no pattern in your blood sugars, take this test to find the cause. Circle your answers.

Do you have:

• Frequent or severe low blood sugars?	yes	no
• Lots of stress?	yes	no
• Erratic eating (different carbs, different times)?	yes	no
• Skipped meals?	yes	no
• Insulin doses that change a lot from day to day?	yes	no
• Exercise that varies in timing, duration & intensity?	yes	no
• No exercise at all?	yes	no
• Irregular sleep hours?	yes	no

Table 28.1 These areas might be causing your rollercoaster ride

highs are then followed in the next few hours by another low, too much insulin is being used to treat the highs.

What To Do:

- Use glucose tablets or quick carbs for all insulin reactions. Glucose tablets provide the fastest relief and can be precisely measured to avoid overtreatment.

- Eat less carbohydrate to treat lows. For most reactions, 15 grams of fast-acting carbohydrate will bring the low quickly back to normal. Fifteen grams is the equivalent of a cup of milk and one square graham cracker, or two-thirds of a banana, or 4 to 5 ounces of a regular soda. Twenty minutes later, when brain function has returned, retest your blood sugar. Only then decide whether you need to eat more carbohydrate (except when blood sugars are dropping fast and more carbohydrate is obviously needed).

- If you are unable to stop yourself from overeating, keep track of the total amount of carbohydrate you eat. Subtract the carbs you actually needed to cover your reaction and then cover some of the extra carbohydrate with an injection of Regular insulin.

- If you have frequent readings below 70 mg/dl (3.9 mmol), review your insulin doses to determine where this excess insulin is coming from. If you are uncertain about how to change your insulin, contact your physician/health care team immediately.

An Up and Down Lifestyle

People are usually aware of the consistency or inconsistency in their lifestyle. If you are not eating and sleeping at regular times, if your work or school schedule is erratic, or if you are not exercising on a regular schedule, this is easy to recognize. Perhaps you have started a new job, are adding exercise to a jumbled schedule, or don't always eat your dinner on time. These lifestyle demands have metabolic consequences that test your ability to use flexible insulin therapy.

A consistent lifestyle makes it easier to set appropriate insulin doses. If you have an irregular lifestyle and also have variable blood sugars, try creating as stable a lifestyle as you can. After your insulin doses have been sorted out, you can return to your previous schedule, if this is absolutely necessary.

What To Do:

- Start testing and charting your blood sugars and insulin doses before and after meals. Add notes on your charts about stress, exercise, sleep, work hours, and your general health.

- Eat regular meals with the same amount of carbohydrate at the same time of day for awhile.

- Monitor your exercise. Note what kind of exercise has unpredictable effects on your blood sugars.

- If you work an overnight shift, try to keep the weekend schedule the same as your weekday schedule for awhile.

- If you work a rotating shift, it is advisable to stay on a single shift until your insulin doses have been correctly set. Talk with your employer to see if this can be done. If your blood sugar control is poor and you must work a rotating shift, seek the help of your physician/health care team to sort out this situation.

MISJUDGING CARBOHYDRATES

Because half of the daily insulin dose is used to cover carbs, the correct matching of carbohydrate intake to insulin doses is one of the most critical elements for control. Variable blood sugars often come from inaccurately matching injections of Regular with the carbohydrates in meals. There are four areas where these carb problems usually arise.

Measurement Errors

Good blood sugar control is difficult when carbohydrates are not accurately measured. If the amount of carbohydrate in a meal is unknown, it's impossible to give an accurate dose of Regular for it. Inexperience in measuring carbohydrates, frequent eating out where carbohydrate quantities must be estimated, or simply not measuring can all create problems.

If your long-acting insulin tests were good, but your blood sugars vary when you eat, your problem is likely to be poor measuring of carbohydrates. Let's say you use one unit of Regular for every 10 grams of carbohydrate. Suppose you usually eat 70 grams of carbohydrate for dinner and have great blood sugars with seven units of Carb Regular. But one evening you have "70 grams" covered with seven units and your blood sugar rises. You probably miscalculated the carbohydrate in that meal. On your charts, look for a high or low blood sugar related to particular meals, especially when meals are eaten at a restaurant or friend's house, or if you haven't had this particular meal before.

What To Do:

- Review the measurement of carbohydrates with your nutritionist or physician/health care team.

- Record brand names and quantities of all food on your charts to pick up patterns.

- If you eat out often, try eating a favorite meal at the same restaurant as a routine so you can accurately cover it with a certain dose of Regular. On each occasion, record how many grams of carbohydrate you estimated the meal contains and how many units of Regular you took to cover it. After a few times it will become obvious how many units you need for that meal. (Some of the books listed in Chapter 8 are very handy for eating out.)

- Take your gram scale and Appendix A in the back of this book with you to the restaurant. Pretend you are a government inspector or a food critic. Your self-consciousness will be more than offset by your improved control and the extra service you receive from the waiter.

Irregular Meals

Although flexible insulin therapy is great for bringing variety into your life, too much of a good thing can create problems. Eating a varied diet at varied times can make stable blood sugars hard to achieve. This is especially true if your carbohydrate to Regular ratio has never been tested. Also, your free-form lifestyle may have resulted in inconsistent testing.

This variation is easy to spot. On your charts, blood sugars will rise and fall, but more importantly the timing of meals and the carbohydrate in them will vary from one day to the next.

What To Do:

Allow yourself to stabilize by living life more consistently for a few weeks. Avoid foods high in sugar and fat. During this period in your life, eat set amounts of carbohydrates at set times. Adjust your insulin doses while living this consistent lifestyle. Once you're well-controlled, begin slowly reintroducing variety into your life. You'll find you can handle the variety you want more easily from a base of stable blood sugars.

Foods With Different Glycemic Indexes

As noted previously, 50 grams of carbohydrate from ice cream can have a totally different effect on your blood sugar than 50 grams from a bowl of cold cereal. Although you're eating the same amount of carbohydrate, you'll find that your blood sugar rises higher and faster with the cereal.

Fast-acting carbs (foods with a high glycemic index number) will show up most clearly on postmeal blood sugar readings. If you start with a blood sugar of 82, shoot up to 317 two hours later, and are back down to 123 before the next meal, you have covered this carbohydrate with the correct amount of Regular insulin. However, you either did not take your insulin soon enough before the meal or you ate a carbohydrate with a high glycemic index.

What To Do:

- Rate the foods you eat on the Glycemic Index in Appendix B, if possible. If your foods have a high rating, switch to foods that have a lower rating.

- Before eating a food with a high glycemic index, take your Carb Regular earlier than usual to offset this faster acting carbohydrate.

- Experiment and chart. Instead of a wheat or corn-based cereal, try one made from oats or rice. Try Cheerios® or oatmeal, or a cereal with more fiber, such as All Bran® Shredded Wheat and Bran® or Fiber One®. Instead of a ripe banana, try strawberries. Instead of white rice, try brown rice. Chart your blood sugar results with these foods to build your own personal glycemic index.

Unusual Food Effects

Some foods have unexpected effects on the blood sugar. Candies sweetened with sorbitol may raise blood sugars more than expected. Peanuts and pretzels may do the same. Chinese foods and pizza are renowned for their ability to raise blood sugars.

Occasionally, an individual may have a unique response to a food. One person we know had frequent, high blood sugars that were unexplainable until she noticed that they always occurred several hours after meals that contained two or more ounces of cheese. She did quite a bit of experimenting to find that the high was a very specific (and unusual) response to cheese. Research has shown that pizza raises blood sugars higher than the carbohydrate content suggests it should,[66] confirming the experience many people have had with it. Some have noted that pizza that has less fat, such as vegetarian varieties, often will not raise the blood sugar as high.

What To Do:

- Write down all the foods you eat on your charts, not just those with carbohydrate.

- If you suspect that a particular food affects your blood sugar, record your blood sugar readings after you eat it. Compare these readings to other meals with similar amounts of carbohydrate. If you see a pattern of high blood sugars after eating the suspected food, eliminate it from your meals or reduce the amount you eat.

- If you are suspicious of a food that is low in carbohydrate such as cheese or meat, omit it or eat less. Then see if your readings improve.

- If you suspect your blood sugar variability is due to food, get assistance from your physician or nutritionist to sort it out.

STRESS

Stress can be overwhelming at times. Difficult times may occur during an extended illness, the death of a family member or friend, or a problematic work situation or relationship. The combination of several factors may occur at one time.

Stress interferes with blood sugar control in several ways. Stressful events are usually accompanied by disruptions in your normal lifestyle. You may lose sleep, exercise less, and eat more fast foods high in sugar and fat.

Stress also interferes with blood sugar control when the body releases too many stress hormones. Fight or flight hormones help us remain alert and active during dangerous situations. Unfortunately, the hormones also interfere with insulin's action, and cause extra glucose to be produced and released into the blood. Higher blood sugars result, along with the need for more insulin.

Emotions and blood sugars are interrelated. During emotional times, blood sugars usually rise (although in some circumstances they may fall). High blood sugars then cause additional stress hormones to be released, which can magnify the emotional reaction. High blood sugars also can cause changes within brain cells, producing depression and irritability. The result is an impaired ability to deal with the stress at hand.

The challenge of simply caring for your diabetes can cause stress and frustration. During your first attempts at controlling blood sugars, you can become frustrated when good results are slow in coming.

Stress may also cause a person to become very active, even hyperactive. This increased activity may cause blood sugars to fall.

If you feel like a totally different person when you have had a few days off from your stressful routine and your blood sugars are much easier to control, consider carefully how much stress you are under.

Other people often see our stress before we do. Pay attention to other's comments. They are often a good barometer of our own stress levels.

What To Do:

- Practice good eating habits even during stressful times. If you avoid candy bars when life is going well, you are less likely to pick up a candy bar when stress hits.

- Test your blood sugars. During stress, testing and exercise are often the first things dropped from your lifestyle. Testing makes normal blood sugars possible. With normal blood sugars, brain function improves and stress hormone levels are lower. Whatever the source of stress, it can be handled better when blood sugars are under good control.

- Take time daily to exercise, especially when stressed. Moving the feet can do wonders for the mind. Exercise releases endorphins in the brain to help you feel better and handle stress better.

- Be aware that the demands of blood glucose monitoring, counting carbohydrates, and blood glucose regulation can be overwhelming at times. Take a break when you need one. Determine how much time off you need to clear your mind. Take the time needed, so you can come back to your monitoring with new vigor.

- If you feel frustrated by your blood sugar readings or doubt that you can make any sense out of your charts, seek help. Talk with your physician or ask for a referral to someone who specializes in blood sugar control.

- How you respond to stress is largely a learned process. If you note frequent high blood sugars following job pressure, arguments, or bad news, consider learning new responses. Stress management classes are offered by many community colleges and employers.

- Talk. Stress is always worse when carried alone. Share your feelings, worries, guilt and pain with others. No burden is too great to share with others.

Life hardly ever lives up to our anxieties.
Paul Monash

RESEARCH INSIGHTS

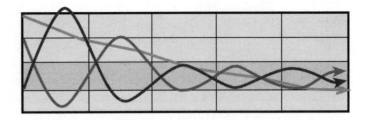

HOW TO PREVENT AND MINIMIZE COMPLICATIONS

29

Complications are a major concern of everyone who has diabetes. This chapter will discuss briefly some of the most common complications, their causes and basic strategies for prevention.

This chapter covers:

- Dangers of high blood sugars
- Why only certain organs are damaged
- Eye problems (retinopathy)
- Kidney problems (nephropathy)
- Nerve disorders (neuropathy)
- Heart and circulatory problems
- Ways to protect against complications

THE DCCT AND COMPLICATIONS

In the Diabetes Complications and Controls Trial, a group of 1,441 volunteers with Type I diabetes were followed for three to nine years. Half were randomly assigned to a "control" group in which blood sugars were *moderately controlled* on one or two injections a day. The other half were assigned to an *intensive control* (flexible insulin therapy) group with the task of keeping their blood sugars as normal as possible using three or more injections a day (or insulin pump).

The intensive therapy group was able to achieve better control than the moderate group, and in doing so also had a dramatically lower risk for major complications. In the process of the study, the DCCT study revealed a linear relationship between blood sugar control, measured by the HbA$_{1c}$ level, and risks for eye and kidney disease. This linear relationship (depicted by the solid line in Fig. 29.1 going from the lower left corner to the upper right corner) means that for any increase in the average blood sugar level, the chance of developing eye and kidney complications become more likely. The same risk is believed to hold for other complications.

Compared to the moderate control group, the intensive control group experienced *less eye damage, less kidney disease, and less neuropathy.* The study laid to rest any doubts that people who intensively controlled their blood sugars have less risk for complications. Any improvement in blood sugar control reduces your risks for damage. The greater the improvement, the lower your risks.

DANGERS OF HIGH BLOOD SUGARS

As seen in previous chapters, high blood sugars lead to serious damage in vital cells and organs in the body. This damage results in complications involving the eyes, kidneys, nervous system, circulatory system and heart. The good news is that research led by the DCCT has also shown that *complications can be prevented by keeping blood sugars near normal.*

Keeping blood sugar levels in the normal range, however, is difficult for most people. People with diabetes who live lives with high stress, severe physical demands, or an erratic lifestyle, must work extra hard to avoid high and low blood sugars. In some cases, normal sugars are not possible.

Note the solid diagonal line in Figure 29.1. This line represents the average risk for damage in people with diabetes over a range of HbA$_{1c}$ values. Half of those with diabetes are above this solid diagonal line. They have an increased risk for complications. The other half fall below the line where complications are fewer. Some "lucky" people have a higher than average blood sugar (farther to the right in the figure) but still avoid most of the damage

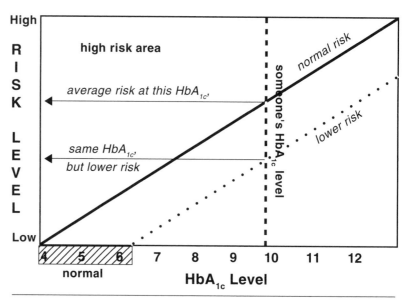

Figure 29.1 Can The Risk For Complications Be Lowered?

(they stay near the bottom in the figure). Why these people with diabetes remain at a lower risk for health damage remains unknown. Let's look at some of the ways to stay in this lower risk group.

WHY ARE ONLY CERTAIN ORGANS DAMAGED?

Cell health depends on a steady supply of fuel from glucose and free fatty acids. These two major fuels are both regulated by insulin released directly into the blood from beta cells in the pancreas. From the blood, an insulin molecule crosses the blood vessel wall and attaches to an insulin receptor on the outer wall of a muscle, liver or fat cell. This attachment triggers the movement of glucose into the interior of the cell, where it can be converted into energy for metabolism, repair and defense.

In contrast to the complicated transport system for glucose, and to the chagrin of many, fat moves easily across cell membranes. If insulin levels are too low, less glucose enters cells, but more glucose is released by the liver and more fat is released from fat cells. So a low insulin level causes not only a high blood sugar but it also causes more fat to enter the blood.

Cells in the muscle, liver, and fat need insulin to receive glucose. The first group of cells that need insulin, those in muscle, liver, and fat, do not become exposed to high internal glucose levels when the blood sugars are high and insulin levels are low. The lack of insulin slows the movement of glucose into these cells, and probably spares them from damage when blood sugars are high.

However, other cells such as those in the brain, nervous system, heart, blood vessels and kidneys pick up glucose directly from the blood *without using insulin.* These cells, except the brain, are more prone to damage from high blood sugars because they become exposed to high internal levels of glucose.

This is one reason why damage tends to occur in these areas of the body, such as in nerve and kidney cells, and in small blood vessels like those in the eyes. They always have their "doors open" to glucose. When blood sugars are high, these cells have high interior glucose levels. The excess glucose makes it impossible for cells or organs to function as they are meant to. They fail to produce key enzymes, fail to repair themselves and fail to transport nutrients needed in the cells.

Nerve cells, are vulnerable also because of their shape. Many nerve cells are extremely long compared to their width. Each nerve depends on

---

Organs Most Prone To Damage:

(Do not need insulin)

- Eyes
- Kidneys

  Nerves

- Blood Vessels

Organs Least Prone To Damage:

(Need insulin, except for the brain)

- Muscle
- Liver

  Fat

- Brain

---

thousands of tiny blood vessels along its path to receive oxygen, fuel, and other nutrients. If one or more of these supporting microvessels become damaged, that part of the nerve is also damaged. Electrical signals in these damaged nerves can then no longer pass, or they pass at a slower speed. This dependence on numerous small blood vessels is why the longest nerves going to the feet are the first to be damaged in neuropathy. Good messaging in nerves also depends on an outer protective coating called myelin. This electrical insulator is also vulnerable to damage from high blood sugars.

Eyes are vulnerable because blood flow to the retina is driven by the need for oxygen. The small blood vessels in the retina (on the back wall of the eye where nerves receive incoming light) have no muscles to limit blood flow. When oxygen is less available (which is worsened by smoking and inactivity) the normal controls on excessive blood flow break down. Blood then engorges the small vessels in the retina where oxygen is low. For instance, when the blood sugar climbs from 100 mg/dl (5.6 mmol) to 400 mg/dl (22 mmol), blood flow to the retina rises to *five times its normal levels*

In Addition To Maintaining Good Control, Remember To:

- Control cholesterol, triglycerides, and HDL
- Keep your blood pressure normal
- Keep your weight down
- Get regular exercise
- Eat varied, healthy foods
- Limit your intake of animal fat and protein
- Eat more seeds and fish
- Eat five servings of fruit and vegetables each day
- Don't smoke
- Have fun!

---

in a short period of time. This excessive blood flow and blood pressure to the small blood vessels in the retina creates an environment highly likely to cause damage. This is especially true when a balancing pressure in the vitreous, the clear gel in the middle of the eye, is low.[71]

Heart damage is caused by the same risk factors found in the general population. But these risks become magnified by high blood sugars. High blood sugars create harmful changes in LDL, HDL, and triglyceride levels, increased clotting, higher blood pressure, and altered blood flow.

People with diabetes have other, as yet unexplained, risks. The standard heart risks magnified by high blood sugars do not explain all of the excess heart damage seen in diabetes. Some possible explanations are discussed in the next chapter.

Brain cells, in contrast to nerve cells, appear to be relatively protected even though glucose is their only source of energy and their "doors" are always open. The brain may derive this protection from the blood-brain barrier and from having different glucose transporters than those found in other organs. Glucose levels in brain cells are normally only *one third the levels found in the blood!*[72] These factors provide a relative degree of protection to the brain.

However, IQ levels were found to drop temporarily in Australian children as their blood sugars rose. When the children's blood sugar climbed to 400 mg/dl (22 mmol), their IQ dropped by 10 percent.[73] Fortunately, this loss of intelligence was corrected when blood sugars were brought back down.

But research in Kansas found that a permanent loss of IQ seems to occur following ketoacidosis that requires hospitalization. Each ketoacidosis episode, with its high blood sugars, in the children studied appeared to cause a loss of just over one point in the IQ. (Although low blood sugars can certainly cause a temporary impairment of consciousness and reasoning, these researchers found no permanent effect on the IQ from severe hypoglycemia in these children.[74] Very severe and prolonged hypoglycemia can cause this type of loss, however.)

Let's look in more detail at the organs most prone to complications.

EYE PROBLEMS

Damage to the eyes is one of the most feared complications of diabetes. Although only two percent of people with diabetes become totally blind, the fear of being in that two percent is strong, as anyone who has had a change in vision can testify. Luckily, loss of vision can be prevented with good control and early detection of eye damage.

To understand how damage occurs, let's review how we see. Vision begins when light is reflected from objects in our field of vision. This light is focused by the lens and cornea at the front of the eye. It passes through the transparent gel, the vitreous, in the middle of the eye on to sensory nerves in the retina. Signals from nerve endings in the retina then travel to the brain where they are neurally constructed into the objects we are viewing.

High blood sugars can impact this normal visual process in a number of ways:

Proliferative Retinopathy

The retina itself is an ultrathin layer of blood vessels and nerve endings. It functions like a screen on which visual images are projected on the way to the brain. Retinopathy is the name for damage of the retina. Damage occurs when abnormal blood sugars, altered metabolism, and vascular changes deliver less oxygen to the retina through its tiny blood vessels.

At first, the damage is minor with no loss of vision. However, as damage to the blood vessels increases, the blood vessels start leaking or hemorrhaging. At this stage, vision is also not usually threatened. But as the oxygen lack becomes severe, growth factors are released that cause the growth of new blood vessels. Unfortunately, these new vessels do not remain in their normal location in the retina, but extend instead into the nearby vitreous (clear gel). These tangled webs of new vessels may be noticed as "spider webs" in the person's field of vision. This situation is quite dangerous because any jarring motion of the vitreous can break open these blood vessels and cause bleeding.

The result of this proliferative retinopathy can be a progressive loss of vision and even blindness. Serious eye problems most often start after about 15 years of diabetes. Over time, if scarring occurs due to bleeding, this may pull the ultrathin retina and detach it from the rest of the eye. The loss of vision is immediately obvious as a "window shade" effect.

Although more than 90 percent of people with Type I diabetes experience some retinopathy, advances in laser treatment mean that most can be helped and can avoid the haunting spectre of blindness. The importance of regular eye exams is clear. These should be carried out at least yearly from the date of diagnosis of Type II diabetes and after the first five years of Type I diabetes.

Macular Edema

Macular edema or "swelling of the macula" occurs when swelling, leaking, and hard exudates found in early retinopathy occur within the macula, the central five percent of the retina most critical to vision. This very small area is rich in cones, the nerve endings that detect color and upon which daytime vision depends. Blurring occurs in the middle or just to the side of the central visual field, rather like looking through cellophane. Visual loss may progress over a period of months, and can be very annoying because of the inability to focus clearly. Macular edema is a common cause of severe visual impairment.

Prevention Of Retinopathy:

Data collected on eye disease in the Diabetes Complications and Control Trial show a direct relation between the blood sugar level and organ damage. For every rise in the average blood sugar level, eye damage becomes both more likely and more severe. Compared to the moderate control group, the intensive control group had *up to 76 percent less retinopathy*.

This data strongly demonstrates the importance of keeping blood sugars as near normal as possible. This will help prevent eye damage caused by the hemorrhaging of tiny blood vessels and swelling of the central vision area, called the macula.

Other steps to preventing retina damage are to:

1. Have a yearly eye exam by an ophthalmologist (a physician who specializes in eye diseases) if you have had diabetes more than five years (Type I or Type II). Early damage to the retina, which you may not notice, can be successfully treated.

2. Check your own vision regularly for danger signs such as floating specks, a spider web, or blurred vision. See your physician or ophthalmologist immediately if you suspect a vision problem.

Cataracts

The lens in the eye is a unique physical structure that cannot be repaired or replaced, but instead accumulates any damage that may occur to it over time. About 90 percent of the material in the lens consists of long stringy proteins laid out like cord wood to allow nearly perfect light transmission. Damage to this precise structure can lead to a cataract.

The most common type of cataract, called a senile cataract, becomes a vision problem in those over the age of 60, although the underlying damage begins decades earlier. A cataract is damage that has occurred to the lens of the eye, which takes in light and visual images just like a camera lens. High blood sugars can turn this clear lens cloudy and diabetes, with its environment of toxic high blood sugars, raises the risk for senile cataract about 40 percent.

Senile cataracts also appear to be hastened by exposure of the lens to ultraviolet radiation from sunlight. Cataracts are more common near the equator and are expected to become even more numerous as loss of the protective ozone layer continues, because the ozone layer protects us from ultraviolet radiation.

Early cataract damage can only be detected by an ophthalmologist. As the cloudiness increases, vision is gradually reduced. A milky film can sometimes be seen on the eye. Vision can be foggy, with halos around lights. Cataract surgery under local anesthesia is the usual treatment. The damaged lens is surgically replaced with a plastic lens. In the United States, cataract surgery is already our most costly surgical expense, costing some $3.2 billion each year.

To prevent cataracts, keep blood sugar as normal as possible and have yearly eye exams, especially if you are over 40.

KIDNEY DISEASE

The human kidney is part of the body's efficient waste disposal system. A healthy kidney cleans the blood by filtering out waste products which are then routed to the urine. Over time, high blood sugars can damage the cells and tiny blood vessels that perform this cleansing. The result is a damaged kidney that routes waste back into the body and releases excess amounts of protein into the urine. Symptoms of kidney failure are fatigue, decreased appetite, nausea and vomiting.

About 30 to 40 percent of people with Type I diabetes, and 20 to 30 percent of those with Type II diabetes, will develop moderate to advanced kidney disease. However, since the damage occurs slowly over time, when action is taken early there is time to prevent the worst of it.

Prevention Of Kidney Disease

In the DCCT, the intensive control group (the group that successfully controlled their blood sugars) experienced *up to 54 percent less kidney disease* compared to the moderate control group (which had less control). So, once again, the best way to prevent kidney disease is to keep blood sugars as normal as possible. Remember that this reduction in eye damage is just due to improved blood sugar control in those with early kidney disease. Other protective measures that are more powerful with later kidney disease are discussed in Chapter 30.

Following these additional suggestions will do a lot toward preventing serious problems:

- Have your urine checked regularly for microalbumin (a simple urine test). This detects kidney disease at its earliest stage when intervention is easiest. This test should be done at least yearly. If any abnormal readings occur, discuss with your doctor how and how often you should be monitored for kidney function.

- Control your blood pressure through diet, relaxation techniques, and blood pressure medications (especially an ACE inhibitor).

- If you have a family history of high blood pressure or kidney disease, discuss with your physician the use of an ACE inhibitor to prevent kidney disease.

- Be alert for bladder or urinary tract infections and treat them early. Symptoms include burning when urinating, frequent urination, cloudy urine, and a strong smell to the urine.

- Decrease animal protein in the diet if you have any kidney disease.

- Remember, once kidney failure occurs, treatment requires dialysis or a kidney transplant!

NERVE DISORDERS

Poor control results in various nerve problems, including pain, lack of sensation, digestive and urinary track problems and impotence. The causes for nerve damage are better understood today than a few years ago, and almost all of these mechanisms start with high blood sugars. In the DCCT, compared to the moderate control group, the intensive control group experienced *up to 60 percent less neuropathy.*

Existing damage is best treated by correcting the abnormal blood sugars. Some damage may be reversible over time. Most of these conditions take several years to develop, so it also takes time for improvements to be seen.

Feet and Leg Problems

When damage occurs in the nerves running down the legs, the result can be as mild as an occasional tingling or as severe as amputation. Symptoms of early nerve damage are: numbness, tingling, burning, or a decreased sense of touch. Sometimes the onset of symptoms is rapid and includes intense pain.

Damage to nerves increases the risk for damage in the legs and feet. When the loss of feeling is severe, injuries to the feet may not be felt. (John Walsh, for instance, had a patient who walked into the clinic after injuring his foot about a month before. He still had the small nail that caused the injury embedded in his foot!) Infection can then set in and can lead to an amputation. When circulatory problems are also present, the risk increases for foot and leg complications.

Prevention of Feet and Leg Problems

Wash and inspect your feet daily. Even small scratches or blisters should be treated with a mild antiseptic soap and an antibacterial salve. See your doctor if you have a minor injury that does not heal within a few days. Don't wait until the area becomes swollen or pus appears. That could be too late!

The following are important ways to care for the feet:

- Keep your blood sugars as normal as possible to protect nerves, sensation , and blood vessels
- Give yourself frequent foot massages to increase circulation. A small amount of moisturizing lotion can be especially good for dry feet.
- Be very careful when trimming toenails. Cut toenails to the shape of the toe.
- Wear soft socks and comfortable shoes that adequately support and protect your feet. Check often for wear or damage.
- Remember that smoking is bad for the circulation and increases the risk for nerve damage.

HEART AND CIRCULATORY PROBLEMS

Many risks for heart problems in diabetes are similar to those for the general population:

- Smoking
- Obesity
- High blood pressure
- Family history of heart or circulatory disease
- Too little regular exercise

A look at the list above should suggest obvious ways to prevent heart and circulatory problems. Some suggestions, such as managing your stress level, will also help you maintain regular blood sugars.

GENERAL PROTECTIVE FACTORS

In the beginning of this chapter, we referred to those "lucky" people who have a higher than average blood sugar but still avoid most of the damage of complications. The reason is unknown why these people with diabetes remain at a lower risk for health damage. Some researchers speculate that the reason is genetic, but multiple research studies show only weak relationships between genetic makeup and the risks for complications. Genetics is not to be ignored, but is not a leading player.

In addition to near normal blood sugars, other protective factors appear to be involved in staying healthy. What are these other protective factors and, more importantly, can any of them be controlled?

Some protective strategies that seen to work are simple. Keeping the blood pressure and cholesterol levels normal is smart. Regular aerobic and strength-training exercise are direct deposits into a longevity account. (They also make daily life more fun and keep us physically independent as we age.) Not smoking is a windfall. Less fat in the diet along with a higher percentage of essential fatty acids from seeds and fish helps. Five servings of vegetables and fruits beats simply eating an apple a day. A body weight near ideal keeps the mortician's thumbs twiddling, as does reducing stress and improving how we react to stressful events.

Health Advantages

The health advantage of some of these interventions is significant. For instance, the MR FIT study looked at risk factors in over 340,000 American men, and found that those with lower systolic blood pressures and cholesterol levels had much lower death rates.[75] Over 5,000 of these men reported taking medications for diabetes. In this subgroup with diabetes, the death rate was between 155 and 242 deaths per 10,000 person-years in those whose systolic blood pressure was above 160 mm of mercury, compared to only 66 deaths per 10,000 person-years when the blood pressure was below 140 mm. If the blood pressure is lowered with medicines that do not themselves cause excess deaths, it is likely that a person with high blood pressure will live longer.

Lowering the cholesterol level has major benefits as well. In this same study when those who had a cholesterol over 260 mg/dl were compared to those with a level below 180, the death rate fell from about 130 per 10,000 person-years to around 62. This assumes, of course, that it's actually the cholesterol creating the excess mortality, and that a particular cholesterol therapy or medication does not itself have negative effects.

A Scandinavian study done with the cholesterol lowering drug Simvastatin actually looked at death rates and risks for heart attacks and strokes in people with diabetes. Although only 201 of the 4,444 participants had diabetes, the researchers found a 44 percent lower risk of death and a 54 percent reduction in the combined risk for a heart attack or death from heart disease in the treated group.[76] From this study, current treatments aimed at lowering LDL levels appear to have a good cost/benefit ratio.

SUMMARY

This chapter has briefly described the major complications someone with diabetes may face. Suggestions are also given on ways to prevent and lower the risk for complications. The most important way to reduce your risk is by keeping your blood sugars well controlled. In the next chapter, we'll look at some of the more important complication mechanisms in detail.

It is no longer a question of staying healthy.
It's a question of finding a sickness you like.

Jackie Mason

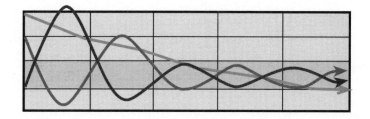

EXPLORING RESEARCH FRONTIERS

30

This advanced chapter is for those readers who are curious about research in diabetes that may lead to better health and longer life. Some of the information is technical in nature. People who are not technically trained may have difficulty in fully understanding the material, but we suggest scanning the chapter for particular areas of interest and for suggestions about changes in health care anyone can make.

Diabetes creates an environment of high blood sugars in which cell and organ damage occurs and the aging process is accelerated.[77] Heart disease, cataracts and other age-related problems occur at an earlier age.

All the complications of diabetes are generated by changes or defects in the body's biochemical pathways. Let's examine some of the research studies and experimental results that point out answers to our question of whether complications need to occur. Keep in mind that there are other biochemical processes *not* discussed in this chapter.

Areas discussed include:

- Sorbitol pathway
- Hypoxia and pseudohypoxia
- Protein glycosylation
- Oxidation and antioxidants
- Homocysteine
- Essential fatty acid deficiency
- Damage to the heart and blood vessels
- Kidney disease

Keep in mind that no one of these processes is totally responsible for cellular damage. They all play a role. The pace of developments, as researchers sort out the importance of each mechanism, has been slow and the reason is simple: complications are complicated. Don't expect any magic bullets. Instead, look for practical interventions that can enhance your health.

The following are ways in which the body can break down and function abnormally due to high blood sugars. Research is underway to test whether medications, changes in diet or exercise, or the use of complementary therapies can prevent or minimize damage. Early results appear to be quite promising.

SORBITOL PATHWAY

One mechanism which causes complications involves the funneling of excess glucose into two by-products called sorbitol and fructose. Both of these by-products rise in the blood along with glucose when control is poor. Their buildup is triggered by high blood sugars and made possible by two enzymes: aldose reductase (AR) and sorbitol dehydrogenase (SDH). AR converts glucose to sorbitol and SDH converts sorbitol to fructose.

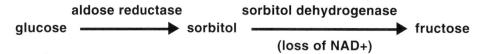

glucose →(aldose reductase)→ **sorbitol** →(sorbitol dehydrogenase, (loss of NAD+))→ **fructose**

As the overactivity of SDH rises, it creates fructose from excess sorbitol. But more importantly, the overactivity uses up critical stores of energy in the form of NAD+. NAD+ energizes many of the enzymes we need to stay healthy. But as SDH becomes overactive and NAD+ levels go down, enzymes that depend on NAD+ cannot do their work. One consequence of this process is the loss of an important protective antioxidant called glutathione.

ATP, Potassium and Sodium Problems

Excess sorbitol also causes myoinositol levels to drop. Myoinositol helps form ATP which, like NAD+, is a source of energy for cells. As myoinositol levels drop, the cells of someone with diabetes lose as much as 30 percent of their energy stored in the form of ATP. The ATP powers enzymes like sodium-potassium ATPase and also calcium-magnesium ATPase that are located within the cell wall.

Each of these enzymes pumps one mineral into cells and pumps another out. Sodium-potassium ATPase, for instance, usually exchanges three potassium ions for two sodiums. This creates a healthy negative electrical charge on the cell wall. But it doesn't work as well when (1) it has less ATP to drive it and (2) it becomes oxidized or glycosylated (see below) in the high sugar environment.

With less ATP, cells have trouble absorbing minerals and charged amino acids needed by cells to build important enzymes and structures. This difficulty creates electrical and energy imbalances and a poorly charged cell. The cell has trouble ridding itself of sodium and sorting out what passes through its walls and what doesn't.

People who later develop high blood pressure and kidney disease will usually first develop a loss of negative charge on cells. In its early stages, this electrical problem can be completely corrected through good blood sugar control.[78]

Vitamins and Minerals

When the aldose reductase (AR) pathway increases in activity, certain vitamin and mineral problems occur. Vitamin C levels, for instance, are low in diabetes, partly because of this activity. These low vitamin C levels can be corrected either by the intake of myoinositol supplements or by the AR inhibitor, Tolrestat. Interestingly, vitamin C supplements, in turn, have been shown to lower harmful cell sorbitol levels by as much as 50 percent.[79]

Several minerals are lost from the body in direct proportion to the blood sugar level. They may also be displaced from their normal locations inside or outside the cell. The higher the blood sugar, the lower the levels of these important minerals. For example, levels of the mineral magnesium are often low in diabetes. As blood sugar levels rise, cell levels of magnesium, myoinositol, NAD+ and ATP drop. Hundreds of enzymes in the cell depend on having these elements do their work. About 400 of the 2,400 enzymes in the body depend on magnesium to work well. With the lower levels of these elements, cells fail to thrive.

Zinc, a mineral cofactor required by many protein-producing enzymes, is also lost from the body in increasing amounts as the blood sugar rises. Low concentrations of key amino acids, combined with excess losses of magnesium, vitamin C and zinc, create defective enzymes and cell membranes. The impact on blood vessels, for example, appears as weakened, stiff and leaky walls.

Work is ongoing with a variety of supplements and new drugs to see if they will protect against these problems found in diabetes, and not create problems themselves. Myoinositol, ATP and NAD+ levels can be increased with drugs called aldose reductase (AR) inhibitors and by sorbitol dehydrogenase (SDH) inhibitors. Although less powerful than AR and SDH inhibitors, supplements of myoinositol, other bioflavanoids, and vitamin C have shown some success in reducing damage when the AR pathway is overactive.

HYPOXIA AND PSEUDOHYPOXIA

A recent theory about cells which exhibit false oxygen deprivation, called pseudohypoxia, is helping to explain many of the observed effects of diabetes. Researchers in St. Louis, Missouri; Nagoya, Japan; Aarhus, Denmark; and Antwerp, Belguim collaborated to develop the theory.[80] Studies of pseudohypoxia suggest several strategies by which damage from high blood sugars might be reduced.

Hypoxia means oxygen deprivation. The theory of pseudohypoxia was explained at the 1993 American Diabetes Association Conference by Ronald Tilton, Ph.D., of Washington University School of Medicine.

In simple terms, the theory holds that exposure to high blood sugar for periods longer than four or five hours causes blood vessels to dilate and blood flow to increase. These changes are very similar to what happens when cells lack oxygen (as was mentioned in an earlier chapter explaining why the retina is vulnerable to damage). Although oxygen *is not lacking*, the metabolism of the cells changes as if it were, hence the name. Cells that act as though they are not getting oxygen may worsen conditions such as angina and heart disease.

Psuedohypoxia, or false oxygen deprivation, may also affect nerves which depend on an oxygen supply delivered through blood vessels that are smaller in diameter than a single red blood cell. Psuedohypoxia also may contribute to proliferative retinopathy where abnormal blood vessel growth is thought to be triggered by a lack of oxygen.

The theory of pseudohypoxia expands on the theory of the aldose reductase pathway (see above) as a mechanism for damage. Aldose reductase has its critics,[81, 82] but, many of the changes suggested by the pseudohypoxia theory have been tested and appear to have merit.

To review, excess conversion of sorbitol to fructose causes cells to develop a lower electrical charge, much like a weak battery in a toy. A series of destructive changes ensues: dilation of blood vessels, increased blood pressure in small blood vessels (called microvascular hypertension), more free radical production, more oxidation, leaky blood vessels, loss of sodium-potassium ATPase activity (linked to high blood pressure, kidney disease, insulin resistance, and other problems), accumulation of fructose (which leads to excess protein glycosylation, described below), gradual hardening of blood vessels and loss of blood flow, and weakening of the heart. Fortunately, almost all of these damage mechanisms are potential sites for drug and biochemical interventions.

PROTEIN GLYCOSYLATION

Even when blood sugars are normal, some glucose molecules attach themselves to nearby proteins. But as blood sugars rise, more glucose attaches to more structural proteins, enzymes, and even DNA. This sugar-pairing process, called glycosylation, creates proteins with defective

---

Bottom Line: Exercise helps to prevent oxygen deprivation and reduce complications.

structures. Glucose is the most abundant sugar in the body and uncontrolled diabetes causes more of it to attach to proteins and eventually form irreversible cross-links between proteins.

Proteins and enzymes need precise structures to do their work, but unfortunately, glycosylation damages these structures.[83] As sugar attaches to proteins, the sugar-paired proteins become weaker as building blocks and perform less work. The abnormal attachment of glucose to proteins is thought to contribute to nerve damage,[84] eye damage,[85] kidney damage, arthritis, DNA damage, cataracts, high blood pressure and blood vessel damage.

Arthritis and joint problems are more common with diabetes.[86] This link between high blood sugars and joint problems is probably due to the glycosylation of collagen, a structural protein in joints. Sugar-attached collagen leads to roughening and thickening of tendons and joint surfaces. Another cause for joint problems may be the excess levels of superoxide free radicals found in poorly controlled diabetes.[87] Superoxide radicals are created *at much faster rates* by sugar-paired proteins, and these superoxide radicals prefer collagen as the target for their destruction. Worsening of joint problems results.

Glucose has even been shown to attach to **DNA** in bacteria and is thought to do the same in humans.[83] The significance of this is unknown. However, damage to mitochondrial DNA is thought to be one cause of aging[88] and may be a cause of Type II diabetes.[89]

Long-Term Blood Sugar Checks

The fructosamine and HbA$_{1c}$ tests provide a good way to measure blood sugar control.

The HbA$_{1c}$ or glycosylated hemoglobin test measures how much hemoglobin (a protein in red cells with a 10-week lifespan) has been glycosylated in the past eight weeks. The more glucose in the blood during the test period, the more glucose that will have attached (glycosylated) to hemoglobin.

The fructosamine test measures how much glucose is attached to a wider range of proteins, not just to the hemoglobin that carries oxygen.

Because glycosylation (due to blood sugar highs) damages the structure of these proteins, these two tests also provide a picture of how much internal damage may have occurred to other proteins in the body.

Cataracts are another by-product of sugar attachment. The lens at the front of the eye allows us to see the world. About 98 percent of the dry weight of the lens is made of straight proteins arranged to let light pass through, much like an open venetian blind. These structural proteins can become damaged, either by oxidizing radiation found in sunlight (which is why sunglasses and antioxidants are used to prevent cataracts), or by glycosylation. On average, cataracts occur 10 to 15 years earlier in people with poorly-controlled diabetes. Another factor that doubles the risk of cataracts is smoking, partly from the increased oxidation created by the toxic compounds found in smoke.

Basement membrane is another structure vulnerable to glycosylation. Normal basement membrane is a thin, supporting matrix of protein found in small blood vessel walls, kidneys and eyes. When blood sugars are high, these membranes thicken, partly as a result of excess sugar attachment. These stiffer membranes allow large proteins to leak through. As blood vessels stiffen, the blood pressure rises. This abnormal thickening can be reversed by bringing the blood sugars under better control.

ACCELERATED AGING

The glycosylation of proteins is bad enough. However, in a process called the Maillard reaction, two nearby sugar-paired proteins become cross-linked to form permanently damaged structures. These damaged structures are called Advanced Glycosylation Endproducts or AGEs. AGE is a terrific acronym because, as the name implies, it is thought to cause accelerated aging.

LDL, often called "bad" cholesterol, is not really that bad. Only after its structure becomes modified by oxidation or glycosylation does it become bad and start to block blood vessels. AGE-LDL (that's LDL which has AGEs in its protein structure) is found at extremely high levels in people who have both diabetes and kidney disease. In one study, a control group without diabetes was found to have only 109 units of AGE per milligram of lipid (fat). In people who had both diabetes and advanced kidney disease 30 times these amounts, 3,270 units were present.[90] Kidney disease is associated with far higher rates of oxidation, glycosylation of proteins, and the formation of AGEs. There is also an exceedingly high rate of heart disease.

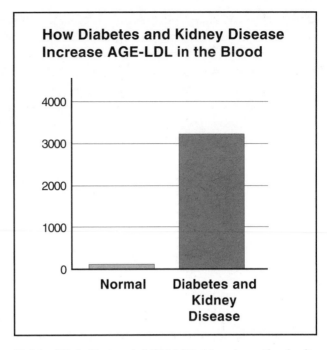

Table 30.1 Normal AGE-LDL Level on the Left.

The dramatic rise in AGE-LDL also keeps cells that line the blood vessels from forming nitric oxide. Nitric oxide is needed to help blood vessels relax and to prevent the growth of cells within the blood vessel wall.[91] Excess cell growth and the presence of abnormal protein structures within kidney cells and blood vessels are believed to be major contributors to kidney disease. These same factors might account for some of the higher risk for heart disease that accompanies kidney disease.[92]

In nerves, abnormal nerve structures created by glycosylation are believed to trigger an attack by the immune system. Such an attack causes nerve damage. When AGEs are present in myelin, the protective outer coating of nerves, they are nine times more likely to start an attack by the immune system.[84]

Possible Remedies

Researchers are working on a drug called aminoguanidine to stop glycosylation before AGEs are formed. One problem in the use of aminoguanidine is its ability to raise histamine levels in a small number of susceptible individuals[93] and possibly create a severe medical emergency. In less toxic amounts, the released histamine may increase the leakage of proteins through blood vessels. This leakage could worsen certain complications like kidney disease or macular edema (swelling of the retina's central vision area).

Another way to decrease the sugar attachment of glycosylation is the use of D-lysine, a biologically inactive form of the amino acid L-lysine. Of the 23 amino acids that make up proteins, L-lysine is a primary target for glycosylation. Researchers have been able to decrease glycosylation in animals by giving them D-lysine.[94] No studies have been done in humans and the long-term effects of this treatment are still unknown.

Glycosylation increases whenever there is more oxidation, the destructive process discussed next. Oxidation appears to trigger the formation of permanently cross-linked AGEs. Fortunately, much more is known about how to prevent oxidation than how to prevent

Bottom Line: The glycosylation of proteins can be inhibited by antioxidants, aminoguanidine (Pimagedine), aspirin, and D-lysine, the inactive form of the amino acid L-lysine.

glycosylation. In a promising development, researchers at the University of South Carolina showed that sugar-attached proteins can be reduced with antioxidants. The study concluded that, "It has always been puzzling that...there are patients in poor glycemic control who appear resistant to complications....The solution to this riddle may lie in the relationship between glycation and oxidation and differences in oxidative stress among diabetes patients." [95]

OXIDATION

Oxidation is a destructive process which everyone is exposed to. Oxygen is critical for the conversion of fuels like glucose and fat into energy, but it can also cause unwanted oxidation. Some two percent of the oxygen used by the body generates free radicals, which attack healthy molecules. These aggressors do not follow the normal rules of metabolism but instead create "rust" in the body. Free radicals are generated in harmful environments such as smoking, smog, excess solar radiation—and diabetes. The process intensifies and becomes more destructive when blood sugars are high. In a healthy person the process is normally kept in balance with antioxidants.

The molecules from which we're made require stability. This stability occurs only when molecules have *paired* electrons orbiting them. Free radicals, in contrast, contain an unpaired electron. With an unpaired electron, molecules become very unstable until they give this unpaired electron to a neighboring molecule or steal one from another molecule. This transfer process takes place in millionths of a second, leaving behind a severed or damaged molecule.

As this unpaired electron is passed from molecule to molecule, a chain-reaction of destructive molecular dominos occurs. Any molecule with an unpaired electron becomes a temporary free radical and will cause damage and fragmentation in a random fashion. This random destruction continues until the electron is again balanced. The balancing agents are known as antioxidants.

Free radicals destroy cell structures. Any fatty acid, protein, or enzyme which comes in contact with a free radical may have its structure crippled or broken. Bruce N. Ames of the University of California at Berkeley estimates that the DNA within each human cell takes 10,000 direct hits from free radicals each day. These free radicals often start the process of protein cross-linking that generates Advanced Glycosylation Endproducts (AGEs) mentioned in the last section. Free radicals are thought to contribute to cancer and aging,[96] and to be a factor in several types of brain damage, including that caused by very severe insulin reactions (luckily rare).[97, 98]

Natural repair mechanisms undo damage by free radicals. But as cells spend more time and energy on repairs, they spend less on other processes essential to health. An individual's ability to prevent free radical damage is thought to play a major role in both health and lifespan.

ANTIOXIDANTS

Antioxidants, a varied group of vitamins and mineral-containing enzymes, disarm free radicals. The most widely known are vitamins C, E and beta carotene. Other important members of the antioxidant family include superoxide dismutase, quercetin, glutathione, selenium, ginkgo biloba and lipoic acid. These and other molecules form an organized system that's designed to stop destruction from the unpaired electrons in free radicals. Antioxidants work by grabbing unpaired electrons while remaining relatively stable until the loose electron is passed to more stable protectors in the antioxidant defense system.

Different antioxidants perform different roles. Vitamin C, for instance, is water soluble and deactivates free radicals in the cytoplasm, the water-based fluid inside the cell. A cell deficiency of vitamin C, called "intracellular scurvy," is believed to contribute to the blood vessel damage found in diabetes.[99] Antioxidants such as vitamin E and beta carotene are fat soluble. These protect fat within cell membranes and fat-based structures such as LDL and blood cholesterol.

Vitamin E

Several studies have been done in the general population that show how important antioxidants are to health. In one population survey in Europe, higher serum vitamin E levels appeared to reduce the risk of angina. A low level of serum vitamin E was a better predictor of angina in this study than serum cholesterol, hypertension or smoking.[100] In another major study conducted in 16 European countries, Swiss researchers concluded: "Vitamin E is the most important factor to explain cross-cultural differences in ischemic heart disease mortality."[101]

Harvard epidemiologists examined vitamin E intake in nearly 40,000 physicians and in 87,000 nurses over periods of four years and eight years respectively. They discovered a strong association between the intake of vitamin E (from food and/or supplements) and reductions in the risk for heart disease. Men who took at least 100 units of vitamin E a day were 37 percent less likely to have heart disease.[102] Women who took vitamin E for two years or more were 41 percent less likely to suffer from heart disease.[103]

Vitamin C

Another large study, called NHANES I, followed more than 11,000 United States adults between the years 1971 and 1984. In this study, UCLA researchers, led by Dr. James Enstrom, found that men who had higher vitamin C intake from both diet and supplements had a 35 percent lower death rate.[104] Women did not fare as well, managing only a 10 percent reduction in mortality, possibly due to their lower risk for heart disease. Cancer deaths were also 22 percent lower in men and 14 percent lower in women who consumed more vitamin C. It is not known, however, whether these benefits are associated directly with vitamin C, or with other protective factors found in a diet rich in vegetables and fruits, or with a generally healthier lifestyle in people who eat more rabbit food. And not every study of vitamin C has found that it lowers death rates. The Harvard study just quoted found no association between vitamin C intake and protection from heart disease.

> **Antioxidant Recommendation From The *Berkeley Wellness Letter***
>
> After more than 40 years of research on antioxidants, so little risk has been found, and the potential benefits so great, that the editorial board of the *Berkeley Wellness Letter* recommends an antioxidant supplement for all healthy adults.[107]
>
> They say, "Supplements of beta carotene and Vitamin E seem to have no significant side effects, even in large amounts. Up to 1,000 milligrams of vitamin C a day also produces no ill effects." according to the nationally respected *Letter* (October, 1991).
>
> Their recommendation: an intake of 10,000 to 25,000 units of beta carotene, 250 to 500 mg of vitamin C, and 200 to 800 units of vitamin E.

The respected U. C. Berkeley epidemiologist Gladys Block, M.D. observed, *"In the United States, plasma ascorbate levels [vitamin C levels in the blood] are disturbingly low in major segments of the population, reflecting equally disturbingly low intake. The results of Enstom et al indicate that increased attention should be given not only to dietary sources of these nutrients, but also to the possible benefits of vitamin supplements."*[105]

What led Dr. Block to this conclusion was her own survey of over a hundred research studies that had looked at the relationship between antioxidant intake and cancer. In her meta-survey, she found 120 of these 130 studies showed less risk for cancer when people had a higher intake of various antioxidants.[106] Though her study related to a variety of antioxidants, she found vitamin C levels very low in the general population and these levels are even lower in people with diabetes.

Quercitin

Another study measured the intake of a bioflavanoid antioxidant called quercetin, found mainly in tea and apples. Among 805 men over the age of 65, higher dietary quercetin was associated with a 27 percent lower risk of death. Cardiac mortality, in particular, dropped by 50 percent, probably due to the ability of flavonoids to stop LDL oxidation and to protect the body from already-oxidized LDL.[108]

Beta Carotene

In one double-blind prevention trial, the antioxidant beta carotene or a placebo was randomly given to 333 physicians. Those in the beta carotene group had a 44 percent reduction in major coronary events like heart attacks and strokes.[109] In the Harvard study mentioned above, beta carotene intake appeared to provide protection to those who smoked cigarettes. Another study, however, found a *slightly higher* risk for lung cancer among those who took beta carotene.

SHOULD ANTIOXIDANT SUPPLEMENTS BE TAKEN WITH DIABETES?

Although taking familiar antioxidant supplements, like vitamin C and vitamin E, appears to help counteract free radical damage, there are limits to this simple approach. After balancing an electron with a free radical and disarming it, each antioxidant has to have its own electrons restored to a paired state before it can again work as an antioxidant. When vitamins C and E pick up a free radical, they themselves become weak free radical generators! For instance, when vitamin C or ascorbic acid balances the extra electron in a free radical, it becomes dihydroascorbate or DHA. DHA levels are already high in diabetes. This DHA causes unwanted AGEs to form and is probably a major factor in creating cataracts in diabetes.[110] Simply taking vitamin C would disarm more damaging free radicals, but it could also leave behind unwanted DHA.

Another antioxidant called glutathione helps restore harmful DHA back to its healthy form of vitamin C. Glutathione levels tend to be low in diabetes.[111] One possible remedy might be to take an antioxidant complex which contains glutathione. People without diabetes have been able to increase their levels of glutathione by taking a vitamin C supplement.[112] People with diabetes who took vitamin E increased their healthy glutathione levels by 50 percent with no change in the blood sugar level.[113] Another antioxidant, the trace mineral selenium, also appears to increase glutathione levels.

While the use of large doses of antioxidants over long periods of time has not been thoroughly studied, we can assume that when too much of anything has been taken, it becomes toxic. But the general trend in antioxidant research shows lower rates of heart disease, cancer and death in the great majority of people who have a higher intake of antioxidants through their diet or through supplements.

CAN ANTIOXIDANTS HELP PREVENT COMPLICATIONS?

The question of whether antioxidants can help prevent diabetes complications will likely not be known for several decades because of the complexity of this type of research. But early studies are suggestive. Two of the major damage processes described here—sugar-attached protein (glycosylation) and free radical oxidation—are intertwined with each other in a destructive cycle. In the test tube, some sugar-paired proteins have been shown to produce *50 times* as many superoxide free radicals as non-sugared proteins.[114] The reverse is also true: oxidation creates more sugar-attached proteins!

There's good news though. Antioxidants appear to reduce this destructive cycle between oxidation and glycosylation. In one study of 12 people with no diabetes who took 1000 mg of vitamin C daily for three months to reduce oxidation, researchers found that their glycosylated hemoglobin (HbA$_{1c}$) was lowered by 18 percent. Another protein, albumin, had 33 percent less glucose attached to it.[115] (Yes, this may help lower your HbA$_{1c}$ test. No, it is not cheating if damage is reduced.) In other studies, vitamin E was shown to lower blood sugar levels[116] and to lower HbA$_{1c}$ levels in people with Type II diabetes.[117] By lessening glycosylation, antioxidants appear to keep proteins in better shape, enzymes more active, and lessen the risk for excess oxidation from sugar-paired proteins.

Low Vitamin C Levels In Diabetes

Disturbances and below normal levels of vitamins, minerals, and antioxidants such as vitamin C, vitamin E, and glutathione are found in most studies of diabetes.[107, 118, 119] It has been known for years that people with diabetes have higher than average levels of free radicals,[120, 121] and in general have low antioxidant levels.[122, 123] For example, your body can be low in vitamin C despite a diet that includes the recommended daily levels.[124] One study measured blood vitamin C levels in 22 people without diabetes, in 20 people with diabetes who had no complications, and in 20 people with diabetes who had complications. These results are shown in Figure 30.2. Note the marked drop in the level of vitamin C with diabetes and the even greater decrease when complications are present.[125]

In another study, vitamin C levels were found to be lower in a group of elderly people with diabetes, and particularly in those who had experienced eye damage.[126] The authors of this study proposed that vitamin C becomes a "sacrificial lamb" to the increased oxidation that occurs in retinopathy. The stress caused by excess oxidation is thought to lower levels of vitamin C.

Another reason vitamin C is lost is the fact that the vitamin must compete with glucose to travel within the body. The structures of vitamin C and glucose are almost identical, so they use many of the same pathways for transport. Vitamin C levels in the cell are normally 25 to 80 times those found in the blood. When blood sugar levels are high, the ability of vitamin C to travel inside cells is impaired. Less vitamin C, less protection.

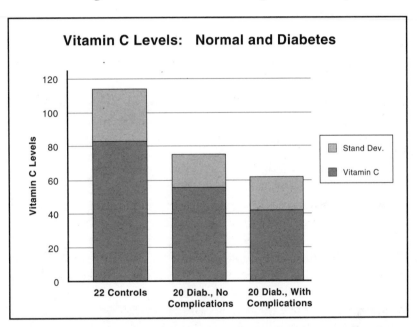

Figure 30.2 Compare diabetes with and without complications

Low Vitamin E Levels In Diabetes

Platelets in the blood provide clotting factors that help to repair blood vessels. Vitamin E keeps platelets from making too much of a major clotting agent called thromboxane. A deficiency of vitamin E increases the risk for clotting, and this can damage both large and small blood vessels. In one study, vitamin E levels in 16 people without diabetes were measured at 295 ng per 10^9 platelets. In 16 people who had Type I diabetes, levels of vitamin E were only 170 ng per 10^9 platelets.[127] In an Austrian study, vitamin E supplements were shown to lower the excess production of thromboxane.[128]

Like vitamin C, vitamin E also appears to protect against glycosylation. One study compared three groups of rats: a normal control group, a diabetic group, and a diabetic group which took vitamin E. The HbA_{1c} level in the normal control group was 2.6 percent. The HbA_{1c} level for rats with diabetes was 7.7 percent. The rats with diabetes who received vitamin E had a HbA_{1c} level of only 5.5 percent, despite blood sugars being equally high in both diabetes groups.[129]

Superoxide Radicals

In 1980, it was discovered that high blood sugars caused more superoxide (oxygen with an extra electron on it) radicals to be produced.[130] When researchers checked the blood for damaging superoxide radicals in 10 people with diabetes and in 10 people without diabetes, they found far higher levels in those with diabetes.[87] When the researchers helped those with diabetes improve their control, superoxide levels were checked again and found to have dropped.

Their results are shown in figure 30.3: people without diabetes on the left, those with diabetes before (middle column) and after (right hand column) blood sugar control was improved. A marked drop is seen in the number of superoxide radicals these people produced once they improved their control.

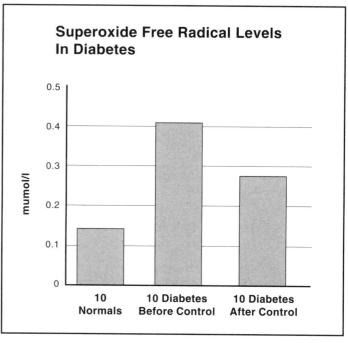

Figure 30.3 Levels before and after improved control

Eye Health And Antioxidants

Under normal circumstances, antioxidants are present at higher levels in the healthy retina than in most other tissues. These higher levels suggest the antioxidants are important for the protection of the eyes.

One test of eye health, called an electroretinogram or ERG, involves shining light onto the retina and then measuring the speed and strength of electrical messages from the retina sent to the brain. An abnormal ERG test gives early warning that damage to the retina is underway. In rats with diabetes, messages from the retina were reduced by 60 percent after only two months of exposure to high blood sugars. In another group of diabetic rats treated with the herbal antioxidant ginkgo biloba, significantly better retina function was found at the end of two months. [131]

Other Antioxidant Research

In German studies, researchers tried various antioxidants (vitamin E, selenium and lipoic acid) in 80 patients with diabetes who had advanced diabetes complications. In the treated groups, the researchers found significantly less oxidative damage and less leakage of microalbumin through the kidneys (kidney disease). They also found some reversal of nerve damage in the legs. The authors of this study proposed that treatment with antioxidants may lead to less damage to the body from diabetes complications.[132]

Whether the higher production of free radicals and lower protection from antioxidants in diabetes actually cause diabetic complications is still not known. Perhaps lowered antioxidant levels are only a minor factor in the damage found with high blood sugars. However, the presence of these conditions appears likely to increase cell damage and compromise health.

Bottom Line: An antioxidant supplement appears to reduce damage. The risk of taking these supplements appears to be extremely low, while research suggests a good possibility for benefit.

HOMOCYSTEINE

Homocysteine, a substance the body normally turns into two amino acids, came into the limelight several years ago. Researchers found some families had a genetic risk for early heart attacks, occurring between 10 and 45 years of age. Some of these heart attack-prone families were discovered to have an enzyme deficiency that created high blood levels of homocysteine.[133]

Later researchers discovered that homocysteine can directly damage blood vessels and is strongly associated with heart attacks, strokes and peripheral vascular disease.[134, 135] Homocysteine attaches to LDL and modifies its structure, much like oxidation and glycosylation do. This modification of LDL by homocysteine seems to accelerate heart disease.[136] One study found that homocysteine levels were four times as high in the LDL of men who had high cholesterol levels compared to those who did not.[137] In another study of nearly 15,000 physicians, those with unhealthy blood levels of homocysteine were three and a half times more likely to have a heart attack than those with healthy levels.[138]

The hereditary enzyme deficiency mentioned earlier is rare. However, homocysteine levels also rise when B vitamins are low, as they often are in diabetes. Excess urination caused by high blood sugars seems to cause the loss of the water-soluble B vitamins. Homocysteine is found at high levels in most people with diabetes who have kidney disease,[139] and in 20 to 40 percent of the general population who have heart disease.[140, 141]

Vitamin B deficiencies also become more likely as we age.[142] One study found a deficiency of one or more B vitamins in 63 percent of healthy Europeans over the age of 65, and in 83 percent of the elderly who were hospitalized for any reason.[143]

A buildup of homocysteine also causes the loss of cysteine, an important antioxidant. In one study, women, ages 20-30, were given a vitamin B-6 supplement, and their cysteine levels rose 50 percent.[144] High levels of homocysteine also lower copper levels in the blood. The activity of some antioxidants depends on copper.[145]

Blood levels of homocysteine are easily lowered with a vitamin B complex supplement. Fish oil has also been shown to decrease homocysteine levels.[146]

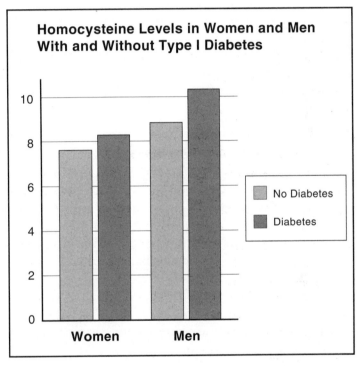

Figure 30.4 Darker bars are people with diabetes

ESSENTIAL FATTY ACID DEFICIENCY

The ways the body burns fats and sugars are tightly linked. High blood sugars can interfere with the metabolism of fats as well as sugars. Fats give cells a form of energy that's easy

---

Bottom Line: A multivitamin supplement containing B vitamins (especially vitamin B6) will help keep homocysteine levels lower.

to store. Some of these fats, called essential fatty acids (EFAs), do more than provide energy. They also act as building blocks for complex molecules that we need for good health. For instance, EFAs, found largely in fish, seeds and plants, are required for strong cell membranes and for the creation of certain biologically-active substances.

Two of these substances are called prostaglandins and cytokines. Along with EFAs, they control the dilation and constriction of blood vessels, reduce inflammation, and provide electrical insulation to nerve fibers that send messages throughout the body. High blood sugars damage the enzymes needed to make EFAs.[147] As key enzymes become inactive, the body makes less of their important by-products.

Cells have an outer membrane that separates their interior from the world around them. These cell membranes are composed largely of fats in the form of phospholipids and triglycerides, together with some proteins and enzymes. Other membranes on the inside of the cell separate important manufacturing sites from the rest of the cell. The membranes themselves contain enzymes that perform functions vital to life. The health of these membranes is critical to the activity of the many enzymes that reside within them.

Examples from among the hundreds of these enzymes in the cell membrane are sodium-potassium ATPase and calcium-magnesium ATPase, both mentioned earlier. The pumping action of these enzymes keeps 95 percent of the potassium and 90 percent of the magnesium inside the cell while similar amounts of sodium and calcium are kept on the outside. This allows the cell to maintain a negative charge. Activities of these enzymes is lowered by oxidation (free radical damage).[148]

Faulty Enzymes and Disease

Abnormal activity of the two enzymes discussed above, and related enzymes, have been observed to occur years before people develop certain diseases, such as high blood pressure, elevated triglycerides, Type II diabetes, and diabetic kidney disease.

Essential fatty acids are critical to the work of enzymes. EFAs also allow red blood cells to flex their way through the very tiny blood vessels that nourish nerves. In poorly-controlled diabetes, there is a loss of the EFAs normally found in cell membranes and in the protective myelin sheath around nerves.

EFAs are more prone to oxidation. Oxidation of EFAs in the cell membranes makes the membranes stiffer, inactivates healthy enzymes, and causes blood vessels to harden. Less production of EFAs in diabetes, together with their tendency to become oxidized, appears to contribute to nerve damage.[149]

Treatment and EFAs

Finnish researchers have shown that improved blood sugar control returns cell membrane levels of EFAs to normal.[150] In early research studies, large amounts of corn oil were used to overcome the EFA defects found in diabetes. Some promising results were seen in the treatment of eye disease,[151] but none of the subjects could tolerate a diet where most of the daily fat intake came from corn oil. In later studies, smaller doses of a fatty acid called gamma linolenic acid (GLA) were given and appeared to reverse nerve damage.[152] A double-blind study followed 113 people with diabetes for one year. Their treatment with GLA improved nerve function on 13 of 16 different nerve tests when compared to a placebo.[153]

Bottom Line: A diet with more essential fatty acids (fish, raw seeds, flaxseed, sunflower and canola oils, and walnuts) may help prevent damage to membrane structures and protect the retina and nerves.

Use of GLA is mildly controversial because it is used to make the fatty acid, arachidonic acid. This fatty acid is believed to be low in diabetes. However, some studies have found it to be higher than normal in diabetes. Theoretically, excess arachidonic acid might contribute to arthritis and abnormal clotting.

Cousins of GLA found in seed and fish oils also look interesting as protective interventions. But the amounts used are important. Eating fish regularly or taking small doses of whole body fish oil may have favorable health effects. But larger doses of fish oil (more than 5 capsules per day) appear to worsen insulin resistance and make insulin requirements rise. Seed oils do not seem to cause insulin resistance and can be obtained in the diet as raw pumpkin, flax, sesame, or sunflower seeds, or as flax seed oil.

Fish actually contain very few antioxidants because they live in an environment naturally low in oxygen. The speed of oxidation or spoiling in fish is well known to anyone who's left raw fish at room temperature for a couple of hours. If you eat fish regularly, you might want to take an antioxidant complex to protect the health of your EFAs.

SATURATED FATS AND INSULIN RESISTANCE

Insulin resistance, also called Syndrome X, is a major health problem in this country and appears to be the most common cause of high blood pressure and heart disease. One reason for this insulin resistance appears to be a higher intake of saturated animal fats in the diet. People with Type II diabetes eat more saturated fat in their diet.[154] These saturated fats are straight molecules that harden more easily at room temperature. Butter is solid at room temperature compared to olive oil because it is a straight fat, while olive oil has a single bend in it. Margarine is made from other non-straight oils, which are straightened or "partially hydrogenated" to create an artificially hard product. When these straight fats are placed into cell membranes, the membranes become stiff. This makes it harder for enzymes and receptors located in the cell membrane to work. The insulin receptor and glucose transporters are two examples. Eating saturated or partially hydrogenated fats makes it harder for them to work.

A higher intake of fat, plus excess weight with an increase in the release of fat into the blood, makes it harder for the body to use glucose.[155] Resistance to insulin rises as we age. But this resistance to insulin found with aging is reversible by eating more carbohydrate in the diet[156] and also by increasing exercise levels. These two steps aso decrease the risk for heart disease.

DAMAGE TO THE HEART AND BLOOD VESSELS

People with diabetes can develop other health problems common to everyone, heart and blood vessel damage being the most important. These problems tend to show up earlier and more often in those with poorly controlled diabetes.

Complications of diabetes involving the heart and blood vessels are associated with high blood sugar levels.[157] This link is less direct than eye, nerve, and kidney complications. Several mechanisms contribute to this excess risk for blood vessel damage. *When blood sugar levels are high, several factors can increase the risk for heart disease:*

Lipid Changes

- LDL or "bad" cholesterol levels rise, increasing the risk of harmful deposits called plaques on blood vessel walls.[158]

- LDL, structurally modified by both excess oxidation and glycosylation, triggers the process that create plaques.[159]

- HDL or "good" cholesterol is less efficient in doing its work to clean cholesterol deposits from blood vessel walls.

- Triglyceride and free fatty acid levels in the blood increase, creating more targets for oxidation and clotting.
- Lipid structures like triglycerides and LDL become smaller and heavier, and form deposits more easily within blood vessels. (Fish oils help lighten them.)

Glycosylation and Oxidation

- Vitamins and minerals that work as antioxidants are lost or deactivated, clearing the way for more free radical damage.
- Glycosylation of proteins causes blood vessel walls to lose elasticity and build up cholesterol deposits.

Increased Clotting

- Blood thickens, making it harder for the heart to pump.
- Common clotting factors rise to unhealthy levels.
- Platelets and red blood cells clot more easily and plug blood vessels.
- The harder outer surface of red blood cells roughens the walls of blood vessels as they pass through.

Other Changes

- Low levels of cell magnesium and high levels of oxidized fat increase the risk for arrythmias.
- Growth hormone levels increase, contributing to a growth of plaque-forming cells.
- Lower levels of L-carnitine, ATP, and active ATP-dependent enzymes may weaken the heart and other muscles. L-carnitine is a transporter for the free fatty acids, and important to energy production in the heart and other organs.
- Higher histamine levels cause excessive leakage through blood vessels.

People who have diabetes develop heart and blood vessel problems much the same way as the general population. However, if their blood sugars are high this environment increases both the risk and the damage. Research studies have pointed the way to possible prevention of heart disease and longer life.

An Aspirin A Day

One promising intervention to prevent heart disease is the use of a low dose aspirin. Studies show a 17 percent to 44 percent reduction in the risk of a heart attack and a 10 percent reduction in death rate due to its blood thinning properties.[160] The Early Treatment of Diabetic Retinopathy Study Group has recommended that people with diabetes at risk for heart disease take one half aspirin tablet daily.

However, aspirin is not for everyone. People who have any history of bleeding, stomach problems, stroke, asthma, or are using other blood thinners like coumadin or heparin, should heed the advice of the American Heart Association's Board of Directors. The board cautions that on the "available data, the clinical decision to use aspirin in primary prevention should be made on an individual basis by a physician or other health care provider."[161]

The actions of low dose aspirin and of antioxidants appear to be complimentary. Although ongoing studies have not yet tested both therapies together, their combined use may reduce the risk of heart attacks more than each used alone.

Bottom Line: A baby aspirin or half an adult aspirin a day looks like an excellent way to lower the risk for a heart attack and possibly to live longer. See precautions though.

KIDNEY DISEASE

Research on kidney disease has also been promising. Kidney disease is the most devastating complication of diabetes. Measurable kidney damage is found in 43 percent of Type I diabetics who have had their disease longer than five years[162] and in 25 percent of those with Type II diabetes for 12 years.[163] Diabetes is the most common cause of kidney failure in the United States. One out of every 100 people with diabetes at any time is in kidney failure (dialysis or transplant).

Kidney damage goes through stages that can be monitored with standard lab tests:

1. **Microalbuminuria** occurs when trace amounts of a protein called albumin begin to leak through the damaged filtering structures of the kidneys. The presence of microalbumin in the urine is often an early warning of kidney disease, but can also be present for other reasons. Normal values on this test are less than 15 to 30 mg/l. The important microalbumin test should be done at least yearly in those who have had diabetes for five years or longer. The test will help those who have had diabetes a relatively short time but have already started to spill microalbumin. As kidney damage progresses, microalbumin spillage will rise above 200 mg/l and be followed by:

2. **Proteinuria** is the spillage of larger quantities of protein. A standard urinalysis will pick up this spillage (normal is less than 100-150 mg/day, depending on the lab). As damage progresses and protein levels reach about 2000-4000 mg/day, proteinuria is followed by:

3. **A rising blood creatinine.** Creatinine is a normal breakdown product from muscle which the kidneys cleanse from blood (a normal creatinine is 1.1-1.3 mg/dl or less, depending on the lab). As damaged kidneys have more trouble cleansing the blood, creatinine levels rise. After a gradual buildup, toxins in the blood reach a critical stage (usually at a creatinine level between 3 and 8). This critical stage requires:

4. **Dialysis or a kidney transplant.** These technologies replace the severely damaged kidneys in cleansing the blood. Transplant organs are scare and the operations are costly. Dialysis is disruptive to one's lifestyle and can cost $25,000 to $45,000 each year.

Reversal of Kidney Disease

One of the authors of this book (John Walsh) started one study to determine the reversibility of kidney damage. He began interventions at an HMO in San Diego in a group of 16 people with proteinuria. At the start of the study, 24-hour urine proteins in the group ranged from 336 to 3,914 mg/day (normal is 50 to 100 mg/day). The study included eight men and eight women. Seven people had Type I diabetes and nine had Type II. The average age was 53 years (range: 24 to 73 years) and average duration of diabetes was 17 years (range: 6 to 29 years).

With kidney disease, protein levels in the urine usually double each year as the disease progresses. A person who is spilling 500 mg of protein per day will reach kidney failure in untreated Type I diabetes somewhere between five and 19 years.[164]

Eating a diet low in animal protein and reducing the blood pressure to normal slow kidney damage. The 16 people with diabetes participated in a multiple treatment protocol. Over a period extending to 16 months, 12 of these 16 people showed a 61 percent reduction in protein spillage into the urine. However, one person had a marked rise of 145 percent in proteinuria and three people had a mild rise of 12 percent. These results suggest that 12 out of 16 people reduced their kidney damage and their risk of needing dialysis or transplant.

Treatment included a low protein, almost "vegetarian" diet with about four ounces of animal products of meat, cheese, or milk per day. Most of the people in this study (11 of 16) received an angiotensin converting enzyme inhibitor or ACE inhibitor. ACE inhibitors have been especially promising in protecting the kidneys. Blood sugar control was also improved with insulin adjustments, diet and exercise. The change in each person's 24-hour urine protein is shown in Figure 30.5.

The Norway study noted in Chapter 29 showed similar improvements in kidney function in people who were at the early stage in kidney disease of microalbuminuria. Their improvement came from simply improving their blood sugar control. Another study done in Italy in the late 1970's also showed early kidney disease could be reversed with good blood sugar control.[165]

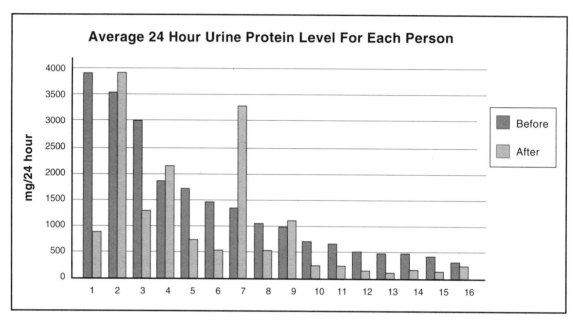

Figure 30.5 Urine protein spillage in 16 people before and after kidney program. Lower values are better. (Normal 24-hour protein values in this study: 50 to 100 mg.)

SUMMARY

These representative studies demonstrate that researchers are gradually uncomplicating complications. Strategies to prevent and reverse diabetes complications will likely be successful only through the use of multiple interventions, with each targeted at one or more of the different mechanisms by which damage occurs. If you have diabetes, it pays to stay aware of these research developments.

When we talk to God, we're praying.
When God talks to us, we're schizophrenic.

Lily Tomlin

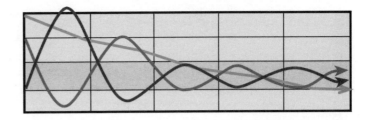

WRAP UP

31

Blood sugar control strategies should be designed to meet your particular needs. The process of learning to control your own blood sugars involves learning more about who you are. In adding flexible insulin therapy to your life, expect to encounter periods where you will meet new challenges. There is no way for you to master this process without learning from a few mistakes.

With any challenging situation like blood sugar control, problems with fine tuning are likely to occur. Besides patience, it helps to have the assistance of a knowledgeable support team.

You are responsible for collecting and recording the information related to your blood sugars. But a health professional's trained eyes can quickly spot important information and patterns in your charts that you may miss. Their experience allows them to help you deal with the questions and problems that arise. How quickly you succeed in your effort at control depends to a large extent on how well you use the knowledge and support of your physician/health care team.

Another helpful aid, if available in your community, is a support group. Support groups are made up of people who have diabetes, their relatives, friends and local health professionals. They provide an opportunity for everyone to catch up on the latest news in diabetes and to help one another with advice and information. Support groups often help their members accept diabetes and deal with it more effectively. Other members understand the rewards and difficulties of having diabetes better than people who haven't shared your experiences.

If you have a support group available, join it for the friendship and information it provides. If none exists, consider forming one. You need no agenda, just the desire to learn and share your experience with other people with diabetes.

We hope the information in this book helps you toward your goal. We learned a great deal in writing it. We tried to keep you, our reader, in mind as we wrote, hoping that we were providing this information in words and ways that would be the clear for you to read and understand.

We offer our wholehearted support for your success as you use your insulin to improve your blood sugars and health. You've already come far, simply by engaging in this process. Our best to you on your adventure.

Glossary

GLOSSARY OF TERMS RELATED TO DIABETES

acetone   Acetone is one of three ketones formed in greater abundance in the liver from fatty acids when glucose is not available to the cells for energy. Acetone, is found in the blood and urine of people with high blood sugars in diabetes and causes the breath to have a fruity odor.

ADA   American Diabetes Association is a national voluntary health organization of professional and lay people interested in research, service, and education in the field of diabetes.

adult diabetes   Now called Type II or NIDDM (non insulin dependent diabetes).

basement membrane   Layers of concentric circles, or chains, of glycoproteins that surround and protect capillary cells in the kidneys, muscles, retina of the eye, etc.

beta cells   Cells that produce insulin; found in the islets of Langerhans of the pancreas.

blood glucose level   The concentration of glucose in the blood (blood sugar). It is measured in milligrams per deciliter (mg/dl) In the U.S. or in millimoles (mmol) or in other countries.

brittle diabetes   A type of Type I diabetes in which the blood glucose level fluctuates widely from high to low, usually as a result of insulin doses not matching lifestyle factors. It can often be improved through a good treatment program, such as flexible insulin therapy or use of an insulin pump.

carbohydrate   One of the three main constituents (carbohydrates, fats, and proteins) of foods. Carbohydrates are composed mainly of sugars and starches.

carb counting   Counting the grams of carbohydrate in the food eaten to determine the amount of insulin needed to maintain a normal blood sugar.

cardiovascular disease   Disease of the heart and large blood vessels; tends to occur more often and at a younger age in people with diabetes. It may be related to how well the diabetes is controlled.

cell membrane   The material that surrounds all cells and acts to retain helpful substances, exclude harmful substances, and allow glucose to pass into the cells with the help of insulin.

cholesterol   A mixture of lipoproteins found in blood, consisting of HDL (high-density lipoproteins), LDL (low-density lipoproteins), and triglycerides.

DCCT Diabetes Control and Complications Trial—a nine-year research study of people with Type I diabetes. Proved that intensive control (flexible insulin therapy) prevents or delays complications of diabetes.

Dawn Phenomenon   An early morning rise in blood glucose levels, caused largely by the normal release of growth hormone blocks during the early morning hours. More likely in Type I than Type II diabetes.

Diabetes Mellitus   A disease in which the body is unable to use glucose normally because of a loss of insulin production or resistance by the cells to insulin.

diabetic coma   Loss of consciousness due to very high blood sugars. (See ketoacidosis)

diabetic ketoacidosis (DKA) (See ketoacidosis)

diabetic ketosis   A serious state of diabetes in which there is glucose in blood and urine, ketones in blood and urine, and possibly some dehydration. This state will progress to ketoacidosis if not treated.

dialysis   A method of washing the toxins out of the blood. Can be either peritoneal or kidney. Peritoneal may be done at home or at a health care center, while kidney dialysis is done at a dialysis center.

exchange   A serving of food that contains known and relatively constant amounts of carbohydrate, fat, and/or protein. The food used in an exchange is usually weighed or measured. The exchanges are divided into milk, fruit, meat, fat, bread, and vegetables.

fasting blood glucose   Blood glucose concentration in the morning before breakfast. Also called fasting blood sugar (FBS). A fasting blood glucose test is often performed to see if a person has Type II diabetes.

fat   One of the three main constituents (carbohydrate, fats, and protein) of foods. Fats occur as liquids or solids, such as oils and margarines, or they may be a component of other foods. Fats may be of animal or vegetable origin. They have a higher energy content than any other food (9 calories per gram).

fatty acids   Constituents of fat. When there is an insulin deficiency, as in diabetes, fatty acids increase in the blood and are used by the liver to produce ketones.

flexible insulin therapy (FIT)   Therapy that uses predetermined blood sugar targets and HBA1c values as goals. The therapy includes frequent blood sugar testing (at least four times a day). Carbohydrate content of food eaten, exercise, stress, and other factors are evaluated to determine insulin need. In early Type II, no insulin or one or two injections, may be needed. In later stages of Type II or in Type I, insulin is delivered by three or more injections a day or by use of an insulin pump.

gestational diabetes   A period of abnormal glucose tolerance that occurs during pregnancy. Precise blood sugar control by diet and/or insulin is required for delivery of a healthy baby.

glucagon   A hormone produced by the alpha cells in the islet of Langerhans of the pancreas. Glucagon raises the blood glucose level by releasing glucose from liver and muscle cells. It is used by injection for the treatment of severe insulin reactions in which the person loses consciousness.

glucose   A simple sugar, also known as dextrose, that is found in the blood and is used by the body for energy.

glucose tolerance   The ability of the body to store glucose. Glucose tolerance is low in people with diabetes.

glucose tolerance test   A test for diabetes mellitus that measures the ability to handle glucose. The person being tested is given a measured amount of glucose to drink. Blood glucose levels are measured before ingestion and at regular intervals up to 6 hours after ingestion. Also called oral glucose tolerance test (OGTT).

glycogen   Glycogen is the form in which the liver and muscles store glucose. It may be broken down to active blood glucose during an insulin reaction, a fast or exercise.

gram   A small unit of weight in the metric system. Used in weighing food. An ounce equals 28 grams; one pound equals 453 grams.

hormone   A chemical substance produced by a gland or tissue and carried by the blood to other tissues or organs, where it stimulates action and causes a specific effect. Insulin and glucagon are hormones.

Glossary

hyperglycemia   A higher than normal level of glucose in the blood (high blood sugar). Fasting serum glucose levels greater than 105 mg/dl (5.8 mmol) are suspect; greater than 140 mg/dl (7.8 mmol) are diagnostic.

hypertension   High blood pressure (excess blood pressure in the blood vessels). Found to aggravate diabetes and diabetic complications.

hypoglycemia   A lower than normal level of glucose in the blood (low blood sugar). Defined by fasting blood glucose value less than 60 mg/dl (3.3 mmol).

insulin   A hormone secreted by the beta cells of the islets of Langerhans in the pancreas. Needed by many cells to use glucose for energy.

insulin dependent diabetes mellitus (IDDM)   Also called Type I diabetes or juvenile diabetes.

insulin reaction   A condition caused by a low blood sugar. It usually is caused by too much insulin or too little food. An increase in exercise, without a corresponding increase in food or decrease in insulin, can cause this reaction. Symptoms vary from nervousness, shakiness, headaches, and drowsiness to confusion and convulsions, and even in severe cases to unconsciousness.

intensive control   See flexible insulin therapy.

islets of Langerhans   The small groups of cells in the pancreas that contain alpha, beta and delta cells and produce glucagon, insulin, and somatostatin.

juvenile diabetes   Now called Type I or insulin-dependent diabetes mellitus (IDDM).

ketoacidosis (DKA)   A serious condition of the body in which there is not enough insulin. Free fatty acids are released from fat cells and produce ketones in the liver. These ketones or acids result in an imbalance in the blood (acidosis). Large amounts of sugar and ketones are found in urine, electrolytes are imbalanced, and dehydration is present. The onset is usually slow. The condition leads to loss of appetite, abdominal pain, nausea and vomiting, rapid and deep respiration, and coma. Death may occur.

Lente insulin   An intermediate-acting insulin that is a mixture of 30 percent Semilente and 70 percent Ultralente insulin.

maturity onset diabetes   Another name for Type II diabetes.

metabolism   All the chemical processes in the body, including those by which foods are broken down and used for tissue or energy production.

nephropathy   Disease of the kidney. No symptoms are present until very late in the disease.

neuropathy   Any disease of the nervous system. Neuropathy may occur in persons with diabetes and be related to poor control. Symptoms such as pain, loss of sensation, loss of reflexes, and/or weakness may occur.

non-insulin dependent diabetes (NIDDM)   Also called Type II diabetes.

NPH   Neutral Protamine Hagedorn, an intermediate-acting insulin. So named because, insulin's action is slowed through the addition of a protein.

oral agent   Another name for a blood glucose lowering agent taken by mouth, such as a pill.

pancreas   A gland that is positioned near the stomach and that secretes insulin and glucagon and many digestive enzymes.

polyunsaturated fat   The type of fat that is liquid at room temperature, unless hydrogenated (artificially straightened). Includes corn, other vegetable and seed oils, and fish oil.

protein   One of the three main constituents (carbohydrate, fat, and protein) of foods. Proteins are made up of amino acids and are found in foods such as milk, meat, fish, and eggs. Proteins are essential constituents of all living cells and form important structures and enzymes. Proteins (four calories per gram) are burned at a slower rate than fats or carbohydrates.

Regular insulin   A short-acting clear insulin crystallized from the pancreas of animals or synthetically made.

retina   A very thin, light-sensitive layer of nerves and blood vessels at the back of the inner surface of the eyeball.

retinopathy   Disease of the retina. Retinopathy occurs after prolonged, poorly controlled diabetes and involves abnormal growth of and bleeding from the capillary blood vessels in the eye.

saturated fat   The type of fat, such as butter, that is usually solid at room temperature. Saturated fats are usually derived from animal sources.

Somogyi effect   A phenomenon (described by the biochemist Somogyi) in which *hypo*glycemia activates the internal counterregulatory hormones (for example, glucagon, growth hormone, and epinephrine), causing a rebound in the blood glucose level to *hyper*glycemic levels.

sulfonylureas   Chemical compounds that stimulate production or release of insulin by the beta cells in the pancreas and/or prevent release of glucose from the liver. They are used in the treatment of Type II diabetes.

Type I diabetes   Results from inability to make insulin due to a combination of unknown genetic and environmental stressors. Also called insulin dependent diabetes or juvenile diabetes.

Type II diabetes   A type of diabetes that is usually found in adults over forty years of age who are not prone to ketoacidosis. The onset is gradual, and the symptoms are often minimal. Patients are often overweight. Type II diabetes is treated three ways: through diet alone; through diet plus oral agents; or through injections of insulin. Also called maturity onset or non-insulin dependent diabetes (although insulin may be needed as therapy).

Ultralente   A long-acting insulin that is prepared using special crystallizing techniques that produce large crystals with small absorptive surfaces.

unsaturated fats   The type of fat, such as vegetable oil, that is usually liquid at room temperature.

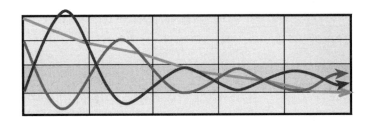

How To Count Carbs Using A Scale And Carb Factors

Appendix A

Few foods, other than table sugar and lollipops, are totally carbohydrate. So the Carbohydrate Factors (percent of total weight that is carbohydrate) for a variety of foods are provided on the following pages. These factors give the amount of carbohydrate in 1 gram of that particular food. To find out how much carbohydrate you are eating in a particular food, you will need to do a simple calculation:

1. Weigh the food on a gram scale to get its total weight.
2. Find that food and its Carbohydrate Factor in one of the Food Groups listed in the following pages.
3. On a calculator, multiply the food's weight in grams by its Carbohydrate Factor.
4. The answer is the number of grams of carbohydrate you are eating.

EXAMPLE

Let's say you place a small apple on a gram scale and find that it weighs 100 grams. You then look up its Carbohydrate Factor and find that it is .13. You then simply multiply 100 grams by .13 to get the amount of carbohydrate you will be eating:

100 grams of apple times 0.13 = 13 grams of carbohydrate

These Carbohydrate Factors give the actual concentration of carbohydrate in foods. For instance, apples are 13 percent carbohydrate (most of their weight is water), while raisins are 77 percent carbohydrate by weight. Breads contain 50 percent carbohydrate by weight. Apple juice and regular sodas both have 12 percent carbohydrate, although the carbohydrate in apple juice is higher in fructose, while a regular soda gets most of its carbohydrate from sugar.

Cranberry juice is even richer in carbohydrates by weight at 16 percent, while grapefruit juice has only 9 percent. A 6-oz. glass of cranberry juice contains almost twice as much carbohydrate as the same size glass of grapefruit juice. Because the cranberry juice contains more carbohydrate, it can raise the blood sugar nearly twice as far as the same amount of grapefruit juice. It will also require almost twice as much insulin to cover it.

Carb Factors For Various Foods

Beverages

carbonated soda	.12	eggnog	.08	milk	.04
chocolate milk	.11	flavored instant coffee	.06	punch	.11

Alcoholic Beverages

beer:	regular	.04	champagne	.01	wine:	dry	.04
	light	.02	liqueurs	.30		sweet	.12

Gin, rum, scotch, whiskey and vodka contain no carbohydrate. With 2 or more drinks, alcohol can lower the normal production of sugar by the liver. Because of the risk of a low blood sugar, no insulin is usually taken for alcoholic drinks. Discuss with your physician/health care team.

Breads & Grains

bagel	.56	french toast	.26	rice, cooked	.24
barley, uncooked	.77	lentils	.19	rolls	.60
biscuits	.45	macaroni: plain	.23	spaghetti: plain	.26
bread	.53	cheese	.20	with sauce	.15
bread crumbs	.74	muffins	.45	toast	.70
bread sticks	.75	pancakes & waffles:		tortillas: corn	.42
corn starch	.83	dry mix	.70	flour	.58
English muffin	.51	prepared	.44	wheat flour	.76

Dry Cold Cereals

All Bran	.78	Grapenuts	.83	Shredded Wheat	.81
Cheerios	.70	NutriGrain	.86	Special K	.76
Corn Chex	.89	Product 19	.84	Rice Krispies	.88
Corn Flakes	.84	Puffed Wheat	.77	Total	.79
Fruit and Fiber	.78	Raisin Bran	.75	Wheaties	.80
granola	.68	Quaker 100% Natural	.64		

Cooked Hot Cereals

corn grits	.11	oatmeal	.10	Wheatena	.12
Cream of Wheat	.14	Roman Meal	.14	Wheat Hearts	.12
Farina	.11				

Combination Dishes

beef stew	.06	coleslaw	.14	potato salad	.13
burrito	.24	fish & chips	.18	spaghetti & meat sauce	.15
chicken pie	.17	lasagna	.16	tossed salad	.05
chili with beans	.11	macaroni & cheese	.20	tuna casserole	.13
chili without beans	.06	pizza	.28		

Desserts and Sweets

apple butter	.46	cookies		ice milk	.23
banana bread	.47	animal	.80	jams	.70
brownie with nuts	.50	chocolate chip	.59	jellies	.70
cakes		fig bar	.71	pies	
angel food	.60	gingersnap	.80	apple	.37
coffee	.52	oatmeal & raisin	.72	blueberry	.34
fruit	.57	danish pastries	.46	cherry	.38
sponge	.55	doughnuts		lemon meringue	.38
candies		cake	.52	pecan	.23
caramel	.76	jelly filled	.46	pumpkin	.23
fudge with nuts	.69	fruit turnovers	.26	preserves	.70
hard	.96	honey	.76	sherbert	.32
jelly beans	.93	ice cream			
lollipops	1.00	plain	.21		
peanut brittle	.73	cone	.30		
chocolate syrup	.65	bar	.25		

Dressings, Sauces and Condiments

bacon bits	.19	olives	.04	pickle relish, sweet	.34
barbecue sauce	.13	pickles, sweet	.36	soy sauce	.10
catsup	.25	salad dressings		spaghetti sauce	.09
cheese sauce	.06	blue cheese	.07	steak sauce	.09
chili sauce	.24	caesar	.04	sweet & sour sauce	.45
hollandaise sauce	.08	French	.17	tartar sauce	.04
horseradish	.10	Italian	.07	tomato paste	.19
mayonnaise	.02	Russian	.07	Worcestershire sauce	.18
mustard	.04	thousand island	.15		

Sandwiches

BLT	.19	egg salad	.22	peanut butter & jelly	.50
chicken salad	.24	hot dog with bun	.26	tuna salad	.24
club	.13				

Fruits

apple	.13	fruit cocktail, in water	.10	persimmons	
applesauce	.10	grapes		Japanese	.20
apricots		concord	.14	native	.34
fresh	.13	European	.17	pineapple	
canned in water	.10	green, seedless	.14	fresh	.14
canned in juice	.14	grapefruit	.10	canned in water	.10
dried	.60	honeydew	.08	canned in juice	.15
banana	.20	lemons	.09	plums	
blackberries	.12	limes	.10	fresh	.18
cantaloupe	.08	mangoes	.17	canned in water	.12
cherries		nectarines	.17	prunes	
fresh, sweet red	.16	oranges	.12	dehydrated	.91
fresh, sour red	.14	papayas	.10	dried, cooked	.67
canned in water	.11	peaches		raisins	.77
maraschino	.29	fresh	.10	rasberries, fresh	.14
cranberry sauce, sugar	.36	canned in water	.08	strawberries	
dates, dried & pitted	.67	canned in juice	.12	fresh	.08
figs		pears		frozen, sweet	.26
fresh	.18	fresh	.15	tangerines	.12
dried	.62	canned in water	.09	watermelon	.06

Juices

apple cider	.14	grapefruit-orange		orange-apricot	.13
apple juice	.12	canned	.10	papaya	.12
apricot	.12	frozen	.11	pineapple	
apricot nectar	.15	lemon	.08	canned	.14
cranberry	.16	lemonade, frozen	.11	frozen	.13
grape		orange		prune	.19
bottled	.16	fresh	.11	tomato	.04
frozen	.13	canned, unsweet	.10	V-8	.04
grapefruit, fresh	.09	canned, sweet	.12		
canned	.07	frozen	.11		
frozen	.09				

Snack Foods							
almonds	.19	marshmallows	.78	popcorn,			
cashews	.26	mixed nuts	.18		popped, no butter	.78	
corn chips	.57	onion dip	.10	potato chips		.50	
crackers		peanut butter	.17	pretzels		.75	
graham	.73	peanuts	.20	sunflower seeds			
round	.67	pecans	.20	no shell		.19	
rye	.50	pistachios	.19	walnuts		.15	
saltines	.70						

Vegetables						
artichoke	.10	carrots		peas	.12	
asparagus	.04	raw	.10	peppers	.05	
avacado	.05	cooked	.07	potatoes		
bamboo shoots	.05	cauliflower		baked	.21	
beans		raw	.05	boiled	.15	
raw green	.07	cooked	.04	hash browns	.29	
cooked green	.05	celery	.04	French fries	.34	
beans: kidney, lima,		chard, raw	.05	chips	.50	
pinto, red, white	.21	corn		pumpkin	.08	
bean sprouts	.06	steamed, off cob	.19	radishes	.04	
beets, boiled	.07	sweet, creamed	.20	sauerkraut	.04	
beet greens, cooked	.03	canned	.06	spinach	.04	
broccoli	.06	cucumber	.03	soybeans	.11	
brussel sprts, cooked	.06	eggplant, cooked	.04	squash		
cabbage		lettuce	.03	summer, cooked	.03	
raw	.05	mushrooms	.04	winter, baked	.15	
cooked	.04	okra	.05	winter, boiled	.09	
Chinese, raw	.03	onions	.07	tomatoes	.05	
Chinese, cooked	.01	parsnips	.18	turnips	.05	

A Glycemic Index For Various Foods

**Each food is compared to glucose which was given a ranking of 100.
A higher number indicates a faster rise in the blood sugar is likely.**

Breads		Fruit		Pasta Noodles	
pumpernickel	49	apple	38	macaroni	46
rye	64	banana	61	spaghetti-boiled 5 min	33
white	72	orange	43	spaghetti-boiled 15 min	44
whole wheat	72	orange juice	49	spaghetti-protein enrich	28

Beans		Grains		Root Crops	
baked beans	43	barley	22	potato, instant mash.	86
butter beans	33	brown rice	59	potato, mashed	72
chick peas	36	brown rice, instant	88	potato, new, boiled	58
frozen green peas	47	brown rice, parboil	44	potato, Russett	93
kidney beans	33	buckwheat	54	potato, sweet	50
red lentils	27	bulger	47	yam	54
dried soy beans	14	millet	75	**Snacks**	

Cereals		Grains (cont.)		Snacks	
		rye	34	corn chips	72
All Bran	54	sweet corn	58	oatmeal cookies	57
Cornflakes	83	wheat kernels	46	potato chips	56

Cereals		Milk Products		Sugars	
Swiss Muesli	70				
Oatmeal	53	ice cream	38	fructose	22
Puffed Rice	96	milk	34	honey	91
Shredded Wheat	70	yogurt	38	table sugar	64

Adapted in part from D.J.A. Jenkins, T.M.S. Wolever and A.L. Jenkins; Diabetes Care 11: 149-159, 1988

REFERENCES

1 The Diabetes Control and Complications Trial Research Group: The effect of intensive treatment of diabetes on the development and progression of long-term complications in insulin-dependent diabetes mellitus. *N Engl J Med* 329: 977-986, 1993.

2 K. Dahl-Jorgensen et al.: Effect of near normoglycemia for two years on progression of early diabetic retinopathy, nephropathy, and neuropathy: the Oslo study. *BMJ* 293: 1195-1201, 1986.

3 K. Dahl-Jorgensen et al.: Reduction of urinary albumin excretion after 4 years of continuous insulin infusion in insulin-dependent diabetes mellitus. *NEJM* 316: 1376-1383, 1987.

4 R.S. Beaser, R.S. Clements, S. Crowell, E. F. Friedlander, E.S. Horton, A.M. Jacobson, R.L. Schneider, D.C. Simonson, and J.I. Wolfsdorf: Upgrading Diabetes Therapy: What every primary physician needs to know. Novo Diabetes Care, pg. 5, 1994

5 A.O. Marcus: Patient selection for insulin pump therapy. *Practical Diabetology* (November, 1992) 12-18.

6 C. Binder et al.: Insulin pharmacokinetics. *Diabetes Care* 7: 188-199, 1984.

7 I. Lager et. al.: Reversal of insulin resistance in Type I diabetes after treatment with continuous subcutaneous insulin infusion. *BMJ* 287: 1661-1663, 1983.

8 I. Lager et. al.: Reversal of insulin resistance in Type I diabetes after treatment with continuous subcutaneous insulin infusion. *BMJ* 287: 1661-1663, 1983.

9 H. Beck-Nielsen et. al.: Improved in vivo insulin effect during continuous subcutaneous insulin infusion in patients with IDDM. *Diabetes* 33: 832-837, 1984.

10 R. Roberts and J. Walsh: The real costs of tight control. *Diabetes Interview* pg. 8 June, 1994.

11 R.S. Mecklenburg et al.: Acute complications associated with insulin infusion pump therapy. *JAMA* 252: 3265-3269, 1984.

12 J.J. Bending et al.: Complications of insulin infusion pump therapy. *JAMA* 253: 2644, 1985.

13 E. Van Ballegooie, J.M. Hooymans, Z. Timmerman, et. al.: Rapid deterioration of diabetic retinopathy during treatment with continuous subcutaneous insulin infusion. *Diabetes Care* 7:236-242, 1984.

14 D. Dahl-Jorgensen, O. Brinchmann-Hansen, K.F. Hansen, et. al.: Transient deterioration of retinopathy when multiple insulin injection therapy and CSII is started in IDDM patients. *Diabetes* 33(1): 4A, 1984.

15 A.L. Peters, R.C. Ossorio and M.B. Davidson: Quality of care for patients with diabetes in HMO settings in California. *J. of Invest. Med.* 43 (Suppl. 2): 256A, 1995.

16 R. Roberts and J. Walsh: The real costs of tight control. *Diabetes Interview*, p. 8; June, 1994

17 NIH, NIDDK: United States Renal Disease System 1993 Annual Report. Bethesda, MD, 1993.

18 American Diabetes Association: Direct and Indirect Costs of Diabetes in the United States in 1992. Alexandria, VA. 1993.

19 A. Lazarow, J.Liambies and A.J. Tausch: Protection against diabetes with nicotinamide.

20 M. Bojestig, M.D. Arnqvist, G. Hermansson, et. al.: Declining incidence of nephropathy in insulin-dependent diabetes mellitus. *N. Engl. J. Med.* 330: 15-18, 1994.

21 N. Perrotti, D. Santoro, S. Genovese et al.: Effect of digestible carbohydrates on glucose control in insulin-dependent diabetic patients. *Diabetes Care* 7: 354-359, 1984.

22 G. Boden and F. Jadali: Effects of lipid on basal carbohydrate metabolism in normal men. *Diabetes* 40: 686-692, 1991.

23 D.M. Mott, S. Lilloija, and C. Bogardus: Overnutrition induced decrease in insulin action for glucose storage: in vivo and in vitro in man. *Metabolism* 35: 160-165, 1986.

24 J.A. Marshall, S. Hoag, S. Shetterly and R.F. Hamman: Dietary fat predicts conversion from impaired glucose tolerance to NIDDM. *Diabetes Care* 17: 50-56, 1994.

25 E. Ferrannini, E.J. Barrett, S. Bevilacqua, R.A. DeFronzo: Effect of fatty acids on glucose production and utilization in man. *J. Clin. Invest.* 1983; 72: 1737-1747.

26 G.M. Reaven: Banting Lecture 1988: Role of insulin resistance in human disease. *Diabetes* 37: 1595-1607, 1988.

27 P. Halfon, J. Belkhadir and G. Slama: Correlation between amount of carbohydrate in mixed meals and insulin delivery by artificial pancreas in seven IDDM subjects. *Diabetes Care* 12: 427-429, 1989.

28 F.Q. Nuttall, A.D. Mooradian, M.C. Gannon et al.: Effect of protein ingestion on the glucose and insulin response to a standardized oral glucose load. *Diabetes Care* 7: 465-470, 1984.

29 J. Beyer et. al.: Assessment of insulin needs in insulin-dependent diabetics and healthy volunteers under fasting conditions. *Horm. Metab. Res. Suppl.* 24: 71-77, 1990.

30 L.S. Hermann, J.E. Karlsson, and A. Sjostrand: Prospective comparative study in NIDDM patients of metformin and glibenclamide with special reference to lipid profiles. *Eur. J. Clin. Pharmacol.* 41: 263-265, 1991.

31 C.J. Bailey: Biguanides and NIDDM. *Diabetes Care* 15: 755-772, 1992.

32 M.S. Wu, P. Johnston, and W.H.H. Sheu: Effect of metformin on carbohydrate and lipoprotein metabolism in NIDDM patients. *Diabetes Care* 14: 1-8, 1991

[33] M. Janssen, E. Rillaerts, and I. De Leeuw: Effects of metformin on haemorheology, lipid parameters and insulin resistance in insulin-dependent diabetic patients (IDDM). *Biomed Pharmacother* 45: 363-367, 1991.

[34] J.P. Bantle et al.: Rotation of the anatomic regions used for insulin injections and day-to-day variability of plasma glucose in Type I diabetic subjects. *JAMA* 263: 1802-1806, 1990.

[35] P.G. Clauson and B. Linde: Absorption of rapid-acting insulin in obese and nonobese NIDDM Patients. *Diabetes Care* 18: 986-991, 1995.

[36] V.A. Koivisto and P. Felig: Effect of leg exercise on insulin absorption in diabetic patients. *NEJM* 298: 79-83, 1978.

[37] J.S. Christiansen et. al.: Clinical outcome of using insulin at 40 IU/ml and 100 IU/ml in pump treatment. Results of a controlled multi-center trial. *Acta Med. Scan.* 221: 385-393, 1987.

[38] J.A. Galloway, C.T. Spradlin, R.L. Jackson, D.C. Otto and L.D. Bechtel: Mixtures of intermediate-acting insulin (NPH and Lente) with Regular insulin: An update. Insulin Update: 1982 edited by J.S. Skyler, Excerpta Medica, 1982.

[39] H. Beck-Nielsen et. al.: Improved in vivo insulin effect during continuous subcutaneous insulin infusion in patients with IDDM. *Diabetes* 33: 832-837, 1984.

[40] G. Perriello, P. De Feo, E. Torlone, et. al.: The Dawn Phenomenon in Type I (insulin-dependent) diabetes mellitus; magnitude, frequency, variability, and dependency on glucose counterregulation and insulin sensitivity. *Diabetologia* 42: 21-28, 1991.

[41] W. Bruns et. al.: Nocturnal continuous subcutaneous insulin infusion: a therapeutic possibility in labile Type I diabetes under exceptional conditions. *Z. Gesamte Inn. Med.* 45: 154-158, 1990.

[42] K. Haakens et. al.: Early morning glycaemia and the metabolic consequences of delaying breakfast/morning insulin. A comparison of continuous subcutaneous insulin infusion and multiple injection therapy with human isophane or human Ultralente at bedtime. *Scand. J. Clin. Lab. Invest.* 49: 653-659, 1989.

[43] B. Zinman: The physiologic replacement of insulin. *NEJM* 321: 363-370, 1989.

[44] J. Walsh and R. Roberts: *Pumping Insulin*: Everything in a book for successful use of an insulin pump. (2nd ed.) Torrey Pines Press, San Diego, pgs. 68-71, 1994.

[45] D. Cox, L. Gonder-Frederick, W. Polonsky, D. Schlundt, B. Kovatchev and W. Clark: Recent hypoglycemia influences the probability of subsequent hypoglycemia in Type I patients. Abstract 399, ADA Conference 1993.

[46] J. Anderson, S. Symanowski, and R. Brunelle: Safety of [Lys(B28), Pro(B29)] human insulin analog in long-term clinical trials. *Diabetes* 43(1): abstract 192, 1994.

[47] C.G. Fanelli, L. Epifano, A.M. Rambotti, S. Pampanelli, A. DiVincenzo, F. Modarelli et. al.: Meticulous prevention of hypoglycemia normalizes the glycemic thresholds and magnitude of most of neuroendocrine responses to, symptoms of, and cognitive function during hypoglycemia in intensively treated patients with short-term IDDM. *Diabetes* 42: 1683-1689, 1993.

[48] A. Avogaro, P. Beltramello, L. Gnudi, A. Maran, A. Valerio, M. Miola, N. Marin, C. Crepaldi, L. Confortin, F. Costa, I. MacDonald and A. Tiengo: Alcohol intake impairs glucose counterregulation during acute insulin-induced hypoglycemia in IDDM patients. *Diabetes* 42: 1626-1634, 1993.

[49] T. Veneman, A. Mitrakou, M. Mokan, P. Cryer and J. Gerich: Induction of hypoglycemia unawareness by asymptomatic nocturnal hypoglycemia. *Diabetes* 42: 1233-1237, 1993.

[50] C.G. Fanelli, L. Epifano, A.M. Rambotti, S. Pampanelli, A. Di Vincenzo, F. Modarelli, M. Lepore, B Annibale, M. Ciofetta, P. Bottini, F. Porcellati, L. Scionti, F. Santeusanio, P. Brunetti and G.B. Bolli: Meticulous prevention of hypoglycemia normalizes the glycemic thresholds and magnitude of most of neuroendocrine responses to, symptoms of, and cognitive function during hypoglycemia in intensively treated patients with short-term IDDM. *Diabetes* 42: 1683-1688, 1993.

[51] K. E. Powell et al.: Physical activity and chronic disease. *Am J. Clin. Nutr.* 49: 999-1006, 1989.

[52] K.J. Cruickshanks, R.Klein, S.E. Moss, and B.E.K. Klein: Physical activity and proliferative retinopathy in people diagnosed with diabetes before age 30 yr. *Diabetes Care* 15: 1267-1272, 1992.

[53] K.J. Cruickshanks and B.E.K. Klein: Physical activity and the progression of diabetic retinopathy. *Diabetes* 43 (1): abstract 84, 1994.

[54] A. Festa, C.H. Schnack, A.D. Assie, P. Haber and G. Schernthaner: Abnormal pulmonary function in Type I diabetes is related to metabolic long-term control, but not to urinary albumin excretion rate. *Diabetes* 43 (1): abstract 610, 1994.

[55] J. Wahren: Glucose turnover during exercise in healthy man and in patients with Diabetes Mellitus. *Diabetes* 28(1): 82-88, 1979.

[56] P. Felig and J. Wahren: Role of insulin and glucagon in the regulation of hepatic glucose production during exercise. *Diabetes* 28(1): 71-75, 1979.

[57] P. White: Pregnancy complicating diabetes. *Am. J. Med.* 7: 609-616, 1949.

[58] J. Pedersen: Fetal mortality in diabetics in relation to management during the latter part of pregnancy. *Acta. Endocrinol.* 15: 282-294, 1954

[59] J. Pedersen and E. Brandstrup: Fetal mortality in pregnant diabetics: strict control of diabetes with conservative obstetric management. *Lancet* I: 607a-612, 1956.

References

60 J. Pedersen, L. Molsted-Pedersen and B. Andersen: Assessors of fetal perinatal mortality in diabetic pregnancy. *Diabetes* 23: 302-305, 1974.

61 K. Fuhrmann, H. Reiher, K. Semmler, F. Fischer, M. Fisher and E. Glockner: Prevention of congenital malformations in infants of insulin-dependent diabetic mothers. *Diabetes Care* 6: 219-223, 1983.

62 J.L. Kitzmiller, L.A. Gavin, G.D. Gin, L. Jovanovic-Peterson, E.K. Main and W.D. Zigrang: Preconception care of diabetes: Glycemic control prevents congenital anomalies. JAMA 265: 731-736, 1991.

63 B. Rosenn, M. Miodovnik, C.A. Combs, J. Khoury and T.A. Siddiqi: Preconception management of insulin-dependent diabetes: Improvement of pregnancy outcome. *Obstet. Gynecol.* 77: 846-849, 1991.

64 J.M. Steel, F.D. Johnstone, D.A. Hepburn and A. Smith: Can prepregnancy care of diabetic women reduce the risk of abnormal babies? *Br. Med. J.* 301: 1070-1074, 1990.

65 M. Miodovnik, C. Skillman, J.C. Holroyde, J.B. Butler, J.S. Wendel and T. A. Siddiqi: Elevated maternal glycohemoglobin in early pregnancy and spontaneous abortion among insulin-dependent diabetic women. *Am. J. Obstet. Gynecol.* 153: 439-442.

66 J.L. Mills, J.L. Simpson, S.G. Driscoll, L. Jovanovic-Peterson, M. Van Allen, J.H. Aarons, B. Metzger, et.al.: The National Institute of Child Health and Human Development: Diabetes in Early Pregnancy Study: Incidence of spontaneous abortion among normal women and insulin-dependent diabetic women whose pregnancies were identified within 21 days of conception. *NEJM* 319: 1617-1623, 1988.

67 C.A. Combs, B. Wheeler, E. Gunderson, L. Gavin, and J.L. Kitsmiller: Significance of microproteinuria in the first trimester of pregnancies complicated by diabetes. *Diabetes* 39: 36A, 1990.

68 L. Jovanovic-Peterson, M. Druzin and C.M. Peterson: Effect of euglycemia on the outcome of pregnancy in insulin-dependent diabetic women as compared with normal control subjects. *Am. J. Med.* 71: 921-927, 1981.

69 G. Perriello, P. De Feo, E. Torlone, et. al.: Nocturnal spikes of growth hormone secretion cause the dawn phenomenon in Type I (insulin-dependent) diabetes mellitus by decreasing hepatic (and extra-hepatic) sensitivity to insulin in the absence of insulin waning. *Diabetologia* 33(1): 52-59, 1990.

70 J.M. Stephenson et al.: Dawn Phenomenon and Somogyi Effect in IDDM. *Diabetes Care* 12: 245-251, 1989.

71 D. Verma: Pathogenisis of diabetic retinopathy—The missing link? *Medical Hypotheses* 41: 205-210, 1993.

72 E. Wallace, M. During and R. Sherwin: Direct measurement of interstitial glucose concentration in the human brain: Effect of changing circulating glucose. *Diabetes* 43 (supp. 1): abstract 144, 1994.

73 E.A. Davis, S. Soong, C. Byrne, and T.W. Jones: Acute hyperglycemia impairs cognitive performance in children with diabetes. *Diabetes* 44 (suppl. 1) abstract 107, 1995.

74 D.D. Fredrickson, D.W. Guthrie, J.K. Nehrling, R. Guthrie: Effects of DKA and severe hypoglycemia in cognitive functioning: a prospective study. *Diabetes* 44(suppl. 1) abstract 97, 1995.

75 J. Stamler, O. Vaccaro, J.D. Neaton and D. Wentworth: Diabetes, other risk factors, and 12-year cardiovascular mortality for men screened in the Multiple Risk Factor Intervention Trial. *Diabetes Care* 16: 434-444, 1993.

76 K Pyorala, T.R. Pedersen and J. Kjekshus: The effect of cholesterol lowering with Simvastatin on coronary events in diabetic patients with coronary heart disease. *Diabetes* 44 (suppl. 1) abstract 125, 1995.

77 A. Cerami, H. Vlassara and M. Brownlee: Glucose and aging. *Scientific American* 256 (5): 90-96, May 1987.

78 H.J. Bangstad, A. Kofoed-Enevoldsen, K. Dahl-Jorgensen and K.F. Hanssen: Glomerular charge selectivity and the influence of improved blood glucose control in Type I (insulin-dependent) diabetic patients with microalbuminuria. *Diabetologia* 35: 1165-1169, 1992.

79 J.A. Vinson, M.E. Staretz, P. Bose, H.M. Kassm and B.S. Basalyga: In vitro and in vivo reduction of erythrocyte sorbitol by ascorbic acid. *Diabetes* 38: 1036-1041, 1989.

80 J.R. Williamson, K. Chang, M. Frangos, K.S. Hasan, Y. Ido, T. Kawamura, J.R. Nyengaard, M. Van Den Enden, C. Kilo, and R. G. Tilton: Hyperglycemic pseudohypoxia and diabetic complications. *Diabetes* 42: 801-813, 1993.

81 R.L. Engerman and T.S. Kern: Aldose reductase inhibition fails to prevent retinopathy in diabetic and galactosemic dogs. *Diabetes* 42: 820-825, 1993.

82 R.N. Frank: Perspectives in diabetes: the aldose reductase controversy. *Diabetes* 43: 169-172, 1994.

83 A. Cerami et. al.: Role of advanced glycosylation products in complications of diabetes. *Diabetes Care* 11 (Supplement 1): 73-79, 1988.

84 H. Vlassara, M. Brownlee and A. Cerami: Recognition and uptake of human peripheral nerve myelin by macrophages. *Diabetes* 34: 553-557, 1985.

85 V.M. Monnier, V. Vishwanath, R.E. Frank, C. Elmets, P. Dauchot and R.R. Kohn: Relations between complications to Type I diabetes mellitus and collagen-linked flourescence. *N. Engl. J. Med.* 314: 403-408, 1986.

86 A.L. Rosenbloom, D. Schatz and J.H. Silverstein: Joint disease in diabetes mellitus. *Practical Diabetology* 11:4-8, 1992.

87 A. Ceriello, D. Giugliano, A. Quatraro and P. Dello Russo: Metabolic control may influence the increased superoxide generation in diabetic serum. *Diab. Med.* 8: 540-542, 1991.

88 A.H. Schapira and J.M. Cooper: Mitochondrial function in neurodegeneration and aging. *Mutat. Res.* 275: 133-143, 1992.

[89] K.D. Gerbitz: Does the mitochondrial DNA play a role in the pathogenesis of diabetes? *Diabetologia* 35: 1181-1186, 1992.

[90] R. Bucala, Z. Makita, T Koschinsky, H. Fuh and H. Vlassara: Advanced glycosylation of the apoprotein and lipid components of LDL reflects the number and severity of diabetic complications. *Diabetes* 42: 119A, 1993.

[91] M. Hogan, A. Cerami and R. Bucala: Advanced glycosylation endproducts block the antiproliferative effect of nitric oxide: Role in the vascular and renal complications of diabetes mellitus. *J. Clin. Invest.* 90: 1110-1115, 1992.

[92] T. Deckert, A. Kofoed-Enevoldsan, K. Norgaard, K. Borch-Johnsen, B. Feldt-Rasmussen and T. Jensen: Microalbuminuria. *Diabetes Care* 15: 1181-1191, 1992.

[93] J. Sattler and W. Lorenz: Intestinal diamine oxidases and enteral-induced histaminosis: studies on three prognostic variables in an epidemiological model. *J. Neural. Transm. Suppl.* 32: 291-314, 1990.

[94] M. Sensi, M.G. De Rossi, F.S. Celi, A. Cristina, C. Rosati, D. Perrett, D. Andreani and U. Di Mario: D-lysine reduces non-enzymatic glycation of proteins in experimental diabetes mellitus in rats. *Diabetologia* 36: 797-801, 1993.

[95] M. Fu, K.J. Knecht, S.R. thorpe and J.W. Baynes: Role of oxygen in cross-linking and chemical modification of collagen by glucose. *Diabetes* 41 (suppl. 2): 42-48, 1992.

[96] R.L. Rusting: Why do we age? *Scientific American* 12: 130-141, December 1992.

[97] B.K. Siesjo: Cell damage in the brain: a speculative synthesis. *J. Cereb. Blood Flow Metabol.* 1: 155-185, 1981.

[98] D. Harman, S. Hendricks, D.E. Eddy, and J. Seibold: Free radical theory of aging: effect of dietary fat on central nervous system function. *J. Amer. Geriatrics Soc.* July vol. 24, July, 1976.

[99] G.V. Mann: *Perspect. Biol. Med.* 17: 210-217, 1974.

[100] R.A. Riemersma, D.A. Wood, C.C.A. Macintyre, R.A. Elton, K.F. Gey and M.F. Oliver: *Lancet* 337: 1-5.

[101] K.F. Gey: The antioxidant hypothesis of cardiovascular disease: epidemiology and mechanisms. *Biochem. Soc. Trans.* 18: 1041-1045, 1990

[102] M.J. Stampfer, C.H. Hennekens, J.E. Manson, G.A. Colditz, B. Rosner and W.C. Willett: Vitamin E consumption and the risk of coronary disease in women. *N. Engl. J. Med.* 328: 1444-1449, 1993.

[103] E.B. Rimm, M.J. Stampfer, A. Ascherio, E. Giovannucci, G.A. Colditz and W.C. Willett: Vitamin E consumption and the risk of coronary disease in men. *N. Engl. J. Med.* 328: 1450-1456, 1993.

[104] J.E. Enstrom, L.E. Kanim and M.A. Klein: Vitamin C intake and mortality among a sample of the United States population. *Epidemiology* 3: 194-202, 1992.

[105] G. Block: Vitamin C and reduced mortality. *Epidemiology* 3: 189-191, 1992.

[106] G. Block et al: Carcinogenesis. *Nutrition and Cancer* 18: 1-29, July-August, 1992.

[107] S.K. Jain and R. Mc Vie: Effect of glycemic control on reduced glutathione levels in red blood cells of Type I diabetes. Abstract 662, American Diabetes Association Meeting, San Antonio, Tx. 1992.

[108] M.G.L. Hertog, E.M.J. Feskens, P.C.H. Hollman, M.B. Katan and D. Kromhout: Dietary antioxidant flavanoids and risk of coronary heart disease: the Zutphen Elderly Study. *Lancet* 342: 1007-1011, 1993.

[109] M.J. Gaziano: Presentation at the American Heart Association 63rd Annual Scientific Session, 1990.

[110] R.H. Nagaraj, D.R. Sell, M. Prabhakaram, B.J. Ortwerth and V.M. Monnier: High correlation between pentosidine protein crosslinks and pigmentation implicates ascorbate in human lens senescence and cataractogenesis. *Proc. Nat. Acad. Sci. USA* 88: 10257-10261, 1991.

[111] S.K. Jain and R. McVie: Effect of glycemic control on reduced glutathione levels in red blood cells of Type I diabetics. Abstract 662, American Diabetes Meeting 1992.

[112] C.S. Johnston, C.G. Meyer and J.C. Srilakshmi: Vitamin C elevates red blood cell glutathione in healthy adults. *Am. J. Clin. Nutr.* 58: 103-105, 1993.

[113] G. Paolisso, A. D'Amore, D. Giugliano, A. Ceriello, M. Varicchio and F. D'Onofrio: Pharmacologic doses of vitamin E improve insulin action in healthy subjects and noninsulin-dependent diabetic patients. *Am. J. Clin. Nutr.* 57: 650-656, 1993.

[114] C. Mullarkey, D. Edelstein and M. Brownlee: Free radical generation by early glycation products: A mechanism for accelerated atherogenesis in diabetes. *Biochem. Biophy. Res. Comm.* 173: 932-939, 1990.

[115] S.J. Davie, B.J. Gould and J.S. Yudkin: Effect of vitamin C on glycosylation of proteins. *Diabetes* 41: 167-173, 1992.

[116] G. Paolisso, A. D'Amore, D. Galzerano, V. Balbi, D. Giugliano, M. Varicchio and F. D'Onofrio: Daily vitamin E supplements improve metabolic control but not insulin secretion in elderly Type II diabetic patients. *Diabetes Care* 16: 1433-1437, 1993.

[117] A. Ceriello, D. Giugliano, A. Quatraro, C. Donzella, G. Dipalo and P.J. Lefebvre: Vitamin E reduction of protein glycosylation in diabetics: new prospect for prevention of diabetic complications *Diab. Care* 14: 68-72, 1991.

[118] J.J. Strain: Disturbances of micronutrient and antioxidant status in diabetes. *Proceed. Nutr. Soc.* 50: 591-604, 1991.

[119] E. Havivi, H.B. On and A. Reshef: Vitamins and trace metals status in NIDDM. *Inter. J. Vit. Nutr. Res.* 61: 328-333, 1991.

[120] Y. Sato, N Hotta, N. Sakamoto, S. Matsuoka, N. Ohishi and K. Yage: Lipid peroxide levels in plasma of diabetic patients. *Biochem. Med.* 21: 104-107, 1979.

References

121 I. Nishigaki, M. Hagihara, H. Tsunekawa, M. Maseki and K. Yagi: Lipid peroxide levels of serum lipoprotein fractions of diabetic patients. *Biochem. Med.* 25: 373-378, 1981.

122 E.K. Illing, C.H. Gray and R.D. Lawrence: Blood glutathione and non-glucose substances in diabetes. *Biochem. J.* 48: 637-640, 1951.

123 C.W. Karpen, S. Cataland, T.M. O'Dorisio and R.V. Panganamala: Interrelation of platelet vitamin E and thromboxane synthesis in Type I diabetes mellitus. *Diabetes* 33: 239-243, 1984.

124 J.J. Cunningham et al: Reduced mononuclear leukocyte ascorbic acid content in adults with insulin-dependent diabetes mellitus consuming adequate dietary vitamin C. *Metabolism* 40: 146-149, 1991.

125 A.J.Sinclair, A.J. Girling, L. Gray, J. Lunec and A.H. Barnett: Disturbed handling of ascorbic acid in diabetic patients with and without microangiopathy during high dose ascorbate supplementation. *Diabetologia* 34: 171-175, 1991.

126 A.J. Sinclair, A.J. Girling, L. Gray and C. LeGuen: An investigation of the relationship between free radical activity and vitamin C metabolism in elderly diabetic subjects with retinopathy. *Gerontology* 38: 268-274, 1992.

127 J. Watanabe, F. Umeda, H. Wakasugi and H. Ibayashi: Effect of vitamin E on platelet aggregation in diabetes melitus. *Thromb. Haemostas.* 51: 313-316, 1984.

128 C. Gisinger, J. Jeremy, P. Speiser, D. Mikhailidis, P. Dandona and G. Schernthaner: Effect of vitamin E supplementation on platelet thromboxane A2 production in Type I diabetic patients. *Diabetes* 37: 1260-1264, 1988.

129 I. Ozden, G. Deniz, E. Tasali, A. Ulusarac, T. Altug and S. Buyukdevrim: The effect of vitamin E on glycosylated hemoglobin levels in diabetic rats: a preliminary report. *Diabetes Research* 12: 123-124, 1989.

130 M. Kitahara, H.J. Eyre, R.E. Lynch et. al.: Metabolic activity of diabetic monocytes. *Diabetes* 29: 251-256, 1980.

131 M. Doly, M.T. Droy-Lefaix and P. Braquet: Oxidative stress in the diabetic retina. *EXS* 62: 299-307, 1992.

132 W. Kahler, B. Kuklinski, C. Ruhlmann and C. Plotz: Diabetes mellitus: a free radical-associated disease. Results of adjuvant antioxidant supplementation. *Z. Gesamte Inn. Med.* 48: 223-232, 1993.

133 J.B. Gibson, N. Carson, D.W. Neil: Pathological findings in homocystinuria. *J. Clin. Pathol.* 17: 427-437, 1964.

134 K.S. McCully: Vascular pathology of homocysteinemia: implications for the pathogenisis of arteriosclerosis. *Am. J. Pathol.* 56: 111-128, 1969.

135 K.S. McCully: Homocystinuria, arteriosclerosis, methylmalonic aciduria, and methyltransferase deficiency: a key case revisited. *Nutr. Rev.* 50: 7-12, 1992.

136 A.J. Olszewski and K.S. McCully: Homocysteine metabolism and the oxidative modification of proteins and lipids. *Free Rad. Biol. Med.* 14: 683-693, 1993.

137 A.J. Olszewski and K.S. McCully: Homocysteine content of lipoproteins in hypercholesterolemia. *Atherosclerosis* 88: 61-68, 1991.

138 M.J. Stampfer, M.R. Malinow, W.C. Willet, L.M. Newcomer, B. Upson, D. Ullmann, P.V. Tishler and C.H. Hennekens: A prospective study of plasma homocysteine and risk of myocardial infarction in U.S. physicians. *JAMA* 268: 877-881, 1992.

139 B. Hultberg, E. Agardh, A. Andersson, L. Brattstrom et. al.: Increased levels of plasma homocysteine are associated with nephropathy, but not severe retinopathy in Type I diabetes mellitus. *Scand. J. Clin. Lab. Invest.* 51: 277-282. 1991.

140 J.B. Ubbink, W.J.H. Vermaak, J.M. Bennett, P.J. Becker, D.A. Van Staden and S. Bissbort: The prevalence of homocysteinemia and hypercholesterolemia in angiographically defined coronary heart disease. *Klin. Wochenschr.* 69: 527-534, 1991.

141 R. Clarke, L. Daly, K. Robinson, et. al.: Hyperhomocysteinemia: an independent risk factor for vascular disease. *N. Engl. J. Med.* 324: 1149-1155, 1991.

142 J.B. Ubbink, W.J.H. Vermaak, A. Van Der Merwe and P.J. Becker, D.A.: Vitamin B12, vitamin B6, and folate nutritional status in men with hyperhomocysteinemia. *Am. J. Clin. Nutr.* 57: 47-53, 1993.

143 E. Joosten, A. van den Berg, R. Riezler, H.J. Naurath, J. Lindenbaum, S.P. Stabler and R.H. Allen: Metabolic evidence that deficiencies of vitamin B-12 (cobalamin), folate, and vitamin B-6 occur commonly in elderly people. *Am. J. Clin. Nutr.* 58: 468-476, 1993.

144 S.A. Kang-Yoon and A. Kirksey: Relation of short-term pyridoxine-HCL supplementation to plasma vitamin B-6 vitamers and amino acid concentrations in young women. *Am. J. Clin. Nutr.* 55: 865-872, 1992.

145 J.C.W. Brown and J.J. Strain: Effects of dietary homocysteine on copper status in rats. *J. Nutr.* 120: 1068-1074, 1990.

146 A.J. Olszewski and K.S. McCully: Fish oil decreases serum homocysteine in hyperlipemic men. *Coron. Artery Dis.* 4: 53-60, 1993.

147 J.P. Poisson: Comparative in vivo and in vitro study of the influence of experimental diabetes on rat liver linoleic acid 6- and 5-desaturation. *Enzyme* 34: 1-14, 1985.

148 M. Kaneko, P.K. Singal and N.S. Dhalla: Alterations in heart sarcolemmal Ca++-ATPase and Ca++-binding activities due to oxygen free radicals. *Basic Res. Cardiol.* 85: 45-54, 1990.

[149] D.F. Horrobin: The effects of gamma-linolenic acid on breast pain and diabetic neuropathy: possible non-eicosanoid mechanisms. *Prostaglandins, Leukotrienes and Essential Fatty Acids* 48: 101-104, 1993.

[150] R.S. Tilvis, E. Helve and T.A. Miettinen: Improvment of diabetic control by continuous subcutaneous insulin infusion therapy changes fatty acid composition of serum lipids and erythrocytes in Type I (insulin-dependent) diabetes. *Diabetologia* 29: 690-694, 1986.

[151] A.J. Houtsmuller, K.J. Zahn and H.E. Henkes: Unsaturated fats and progression of diabetic retinopathy. *Doc. Ophthalmol.* 48: 363-371, 1979.

[152] G.A. Jamal and H. Carmichael: The effect of gamma-linolenic acid on human diabetic peripheral neuropathy: A double-blind placebo-controlled trial. *Diabetic Medicine* 7: 319-323, 1990.

[153] H. Keen, J. Payan, J. Allawi et al.: Treatment of diabetic neuropathy with gamma linolenic acid. *Diabetes Care* 16: 8-15, 1993.

[154] V. Salomaa, I. Ahola, A. Aro, P. Pietinen, H.J. Korhonen and I. Penttila: Fatty acid composition of serum cholesterol esters in different degrees of glucose intolerance: a population-based study. *Metabolism* 39: 1285-1291, 1990.

[155] J. Felber, E. Ferrannini, A. Golay, H.U. Meyer, D. Theibaud, B. Curchod, E. Maeder, E. Jequier, and R.A. DeFronzo: Role of lipid oxidation in pathogenesis of insulin resistance of obesity and Type II diabetes. Diabetes 36: 1341-1350, 1987.

[156] M. Chen, R.N. Bergman and D. Porte, Jr.: Insulin resistance and B-Cell dysfunction in aging: The importance of dietary carbohydrate. J. Endocrinology and Metabolism 67: 951-957, 1988.

[157] J.A. Colwell et al.: Pathogenesis of atherosclerosis in Diabetes Mellitus. *Diabetes Care* 4: 121-133 1981.

[158] F.L. Dunn et al.: Plasma lipid and lipoprotein levels with continuous subcutaneous insulin infusion in Type I Diabetes Mellitus. *Ann. Int. Med.* 95: 426-431, 1981.

[159] D. Steinberg, S. Parthasarathy, T.E. Carew, J.C. Khoo and J.L. Witztum: Beyond cholesterol. Modifications of low density lipoprotein that increase its atherogenicity. *New Engl. J. Med.* 320: 915-924, 1989.

[160] ETDRS Investigators: Aspirin effects on mortality and morbidity in patients with diabetes mellitus: Early Treatment Diabetic Retinopathy Study Report 14. *JAMA* 268: 1292-1300, 1992.

[161] V. Fuster, M.L. Dyken, P.S. Vokonas and C. Hennekens: AHA Medical/Scientific Statement: Aspirin as a therapeutic agent in cardiovascular disease. *Circulation* 87: 659-671, 1993.

[162] H.H. Parving et. al.: Prevalence of microalbuminuria, arterial hypertension, retinopathy and neuropathy in patients with insulin-dependent diabetes. *BMJ* 296: 156-160, 1988.

[163] D.J. Ballard et. al.: Epidemiology of persistent proteinuria in Type II diabetes mellitus: Population-based study in Rochester, Minnesota. *Diabetes* 37: 405-412, 1988.

[164] D.G. Warnock and F.C. Rector: <u>Treatment of Renal Disease in the Diabetic.</u> Upjohn Medical Education Series 11: 6, 1987.

[165] G.C. Viberti et. al.: Effect of control of blood glucose on urinary excretion of albumin and B2-microglobulin in insulin-dependent diabetes. *NEJM* 300: 638-641, 1979.

[166] N. Cohen, M. Halberstam, P. Shlimovich, L. Rossetti, and H. Shamoon: Oral vanadyl sulfate improves hepatic and peripheral insulin sensitivity in NIDDM but not in obese nondiabetic subjects. Diabetes 44 (supp. 1): abstract 611, 1995.

Index

effects on blood sugar   63
  low   206
protein glycosylation   193
proteinuria   205
pseudohypoxia   193
psyllium   170, 171

Q

quercetin   198

R

recordkeeping   28
  Blood Sugar Inventory and Action Guides   33–35
  reasons for   43–44
  Smart Charts   43–48
  with Mellitus Manager   53–55
Regular insulin   15, 74
  mixing with long-acting   87
  Unused Insulin Rule   111–112
retinopathy   4, 21
  proliferative   186
Rule of 18ths   156

S

scatter chart   57
selenium   198
self test
  flexible insulin therapy   22
short-acting insulin   76–77
  absorption of   15
Smart Charts   28
  activity level   45
  blood sugar patterns on   159–160
  content   45–48
  sample chart   44
snacks   64
sodium   192
software
  for downloading meter   55
sorbitol   192
Standard of Care   25–26
stress   47, 116, 124, 127, 179
stress hormones   36, 127–128, 147
sugar   71
sulfonylureas   81
superoxide free radicals   194, 200
Sweet Tarts   123
symptoms for insulin reactions   122
symptoms for nighttime reactions   122
Syndrome X   10, 203

T

table sugar   124

thiazolidinediones   82
thyroid disease   118
Tilton, Ronald   193
Toohey, Barbara   82
triglyceride levels   19
  high   17
triglycerides   80, 204
Troglitazone   82
Type I diabetes   8–9
  causes   9
  prevention   30
  screening for   30
  stages of therapy   11
  symptoms   8
Type II diabetes   9–10
  advantages of flexible insulin therapy   19
  apple figure   79–80
  causes   10, 62
  diet and exercise therapy   83
  insulin therapy   83
  morning blood sugar   17
  prevention   30
  stages of therapy   12, 83
  subgroups of   10
  treatment   10
Type IIr diabetes   10
Type IIs diabetes   11

U

Ultralente insulin   19, 74, 95
Unused Insulin Rule   111–113

V

vanadium   136
Velosulin   87
Veneman, Thiemo   128
vitamin B
  deficiency   201
vitamin C   192, 197–199
vitamin E   197, 199
vitamins   192
vomiting   117

W

weight gain   62, 70, 79–80
weight loss   19
weight, optimum   65
White, Priscilla   152

Z

zinc   192

ORDER FORM

Please send me the following items. If I am not satisfied, I may return any item for a full refund.

ITEM	DESCRIPTION	QUANTITY	PRICE	TOTAL
Stop the Rollercoster	Book on improving blood sugars and diabetes lifestyle.	_____ @	$21.95	$ _____
Pumping Insulin	Book on insulin pump use.	_____ @	$19.95	$ _____

NOTE: The items below come with complete instructions for making sense out of your blood sugar data.

ITEM	DESCRIPTION	QUANTITY	PRICE	TOTAL
The Blood Sugar Inventory and Action Guides (1 unit)	Pocketsize 6-month logbook, pattern analysis, and guide to improving blood sugars.	_____ @	$ 9.95	$ _____
Smart Charts	Checkbook-size, 4-month charts to record diabetes data and determine sugar patterns.	_____ @	$ 8.95	$ _____
Pocket Pancreas	Handy booklet on carb counting, insulin use, exercise, highs, lows, and more.	_____ @	$ 5.95	$ _____
My Other CheckBook	Pocket Pancreas and 4 months of Smart Charts combined	_____ @	$12.95	$ _____
Mellitus Manager® (from MetaMedix™)	Computer software program that downloads, charts, and graphs data from your meter.	_____ @	$79.95	$ _____

Subtotal (add items from above) $ _____

(California res. add 7 percent tax) $ _____

S&H: ☐ Priority Mail $ 3.75 ☐ Bookrate $2.75
(Add $1 each add. item. For Bulk Orders, Special Delivery, Outside U.S., please call us) $ _____

TOTAL $ _____

Method of Payment:

☐ Visa ☐ MC ☐ Check (payable to: **Torrey Pines Press**)

Card # _____ Exp. ____/____

Signature: _____

Questions about your order?
Need it right away?

**Order Toll Free at
1-800-988-4772**

Other calls: (619) 497-0900
e-mail: orders@diabetesnet.com
browse: http://www.diabetesnet.com

Mail this order form to:
TORREY PINES PRESS
1030 West Upas Street
San Diego, CA 92103-3821
or FAX to (619) 497-0900

Ship to:

Name _____

Street _____

City _____ State _____ ZIP _____

Phone Day: ( ) _____ Night: ( ) _____